Urinary Tract Infections, Calculi and Tubular Disorders

John Walls, MB, CH.B, FRCP

Consultant Nephrologist
Area Renal Unit, Leicester General Hospital, Leicester

Published,
in association with
UPDATE PUBLICATIONS LTD., by

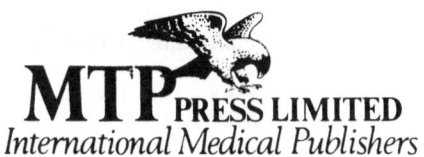

MTP PRESS LIMITED
International Medical Publishers

Published,
in association with
Update Publications Ltd., by

MTP Press Limited
Falcon House
Lancaster, England

Copyright © 1981 MTP Press Limited
Softcover reprint of the hardcover 1st edition 1981
First published 1981

ISBN-13: 978-94-009-8077-8   e-ISBN-13: 978-94-009-8075-4
DOI: 10.1007/ 978-94-009-8075-4

Fakenham Press Limited, Fakenham, Norfolk

Contents

Contents

Preface

This book in the *Topic Pack* series covers some of the commoner and some of the rarer nephrological diseases. Owing to their diverse nature a 'traditional' approach, i.e. one considering pathogenesis, symptoms, signs and treatment, has been used. This inevitably leads to some repetition but the reader should be constantly reminded that apparently trivial symptoms such as frequency, dysuria, etc. may be the clues to more fascinating pathology. In addition, where relevant, attempts have been made to remind the reader of some basic renal physiology in order to understand the results of pathological changes, those changes being illustrated by renal histology, specimens and radiographs.

John Walls,
Leicester General Hospital,

Preface

1. Urinary Tract Infections

Infection of the urinary tract is the commonest renal disease seen in nephrological practice and second only to infections of the respiratory tract in overall clinical practice. With the widespread and early use of antibiotics over the past three decades it was hoped that some of the problems caused by urinary tract infections would be eliminated. However, this has not proved so, as the figures from the European Dialysis and Transplant Association Register (1975) have shown (Figure 1). 'Pyelonephritis' is the

Figure 1. *The main causes of end stage renal failure (from the European Dialysis and Transplant Association Register 1975)*

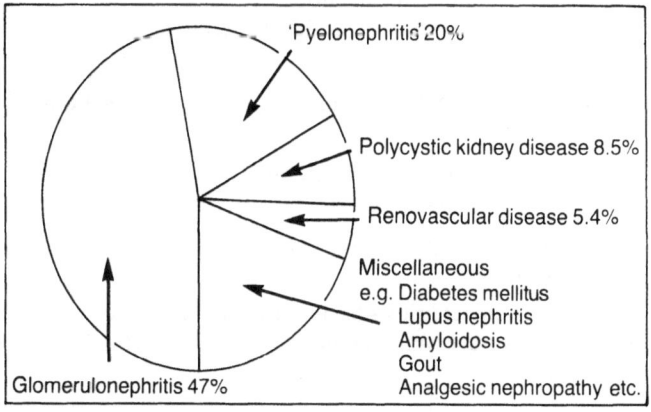

underlying diagnosis in approximately 20 per cent of all patients on regular haemodialysis or transplantation programmes throughout Europe, being second to glomerulonephritis as a cause of end stage renal failure.

In this book on the study of urine Hippocrates (400 BC) recognized stone formation, haematuria and suppuration. Guglielmo Salicetti (12th century) wrote: 'Hardness in the kidneys is produced either after an abscess from which it is gradually scattered, or it begins of itself . . . and this illness is worse than others for it is either not well cured or cured by no means.' The latter half of this quotation could apply to many renal diseases today, particularly to chronic pyelonephritis. In the mid and late 19th century the presence of bacteria in the urine, the suitability of urine for bacterial culture and the occurrence of pyelitis of pregnancy and childhood became increasingly recognized. In the first three decades of this century there were many clinical and pathological reports on acute and chronic urinary tract infections. Today, however, there is still considerable misunderstanding and controversy about the aetiological role of infection in the urinary tract as a cause of renal impairment. One of the problems has been semantic in origin. The use of various terms which are either ill-defined or have changed their meaning often clouds the issue, e.g. cystitis, pyelitis and the overall grouping of chronic interstitial nephritis as chronic pyelonephritis.

Throughout this book the following terms, as defined, will be used:

1. Bacteriuria—any bacteria in urine uncontaminated by normal urethral flora.

2. Urinary tract infection—bacteriuria with or without signs or symptoms of inflammation.

3. Asymptomatic bacteriuria—bacteriuria unaccompanied by clinical symptoms.

4. Acute pyelonephritis—bacteriuria with or without signs of lower urinary tract symptoms but with chills, fever, flank pain and tenderness.

5. Chronic pyelonephritis—renal disease believed to be caused by bacterial infection in the kidney either past or present.

6. Chronic interstitial nephritis—inflammatory changes involving the renal tubules and interstitium due to various causes but when caused by infection synonymous with pyelonephritis.

Another reason for the earlier confusion with regard to the understanding of urinary tract infection was the lack of an adequate definition of bacteriuria.

In a number of studies carried out in the late 1950s and early 1960s, it was established that 100,000 bacteria/ml of urine was diagnostically significant, preferably on two consecutive urine specimens. Since then, many epidemiological studies have had a sound basis and the clinician has a guideline for treatment.

Various aspects of urinary tract infections seen in clinical practice will be discussed. Infections due to tuberculosis and infections seen more commonly in tropical countries, e.g. bilharzia, will not be discussed.

Incidence

Consultations for urinary tract infection in general practice range from 1.0 to 2.0 per cent of all new consultations. A number of studies in which large populations of children were screened have recently defined the incidence and problems of bacteriuria in this age group. Early studies in the USA revealed an overall incidence of just over one per cent. In the UK screening all schoolgirls between the age of 5 and 11 years in two major cities showed a prevalence of 1.8 per cent. Another study, using similar techniques, showed that there was an increasing prevalence from 4 to 11 years of age of 1.4 to 2.5 per cent in schoolgirls, but the prevalence in boys of the same age was only 0.2 per cent. A similar sex difference was noted in hospital admissions for urinary tract infections in Sweden, accounting for 3 per cent of girls and only 1.1 per cent of boys.

In non-pregnant females the incidence of urinary tract infection rises after childhood to around 6 per cent during the sexually active years. The role of sexual intercourse, which will be discussed later, is further highlighted by a 12-fold higher incidence in the general female population compared with nuns. A further increase to 10 per cent occurs after the fifth and sixth decade. Pregnancy increases the incidence to 12 or 13 per cent. The overall incidence in women increases with such factors as age, parity, the presence of sickle cell trait and lower socioeconomic classes.

Urinary tract infection is relatively uncommon in males, until the age of 45 years, when there is an increase to 2 or 3 per cent in the next three decades, presumably due to an increasing incidence of abnormalities in the urinary tract, e.g., prostatic hypertrophy.

Methods of Urine Collection

As the diagnosis of urinary tract infection depends on the demonstration of the causative organism in a urine specimen, the collection of such specimens and the avoidance of contamination is of paramount importance. It was common practice many years ago to obtain a urine specimen by catheterization under supposedly sterile conditions. However, because of the known risks of instrumentation of the bladder and the subsequent development of urinary tract infection, this method should be avoided. Other methods are:

1. The midstream specimen of urine (MSU). The distal portion of the urethra in both males and females is colonized with bacteria, and before a urine specimen is obtained it is necessary to flush these away with the initial quantity of urine passed during micturition. In males this is relatively simple, but in females careful preparation is necessary. After labial separation the vulva should be washed with soap solution or sterile saline before the midstream urine specimen is obtained. In this manner, the contamination rate will be reduced to as low as one per cent.

2. Suprapubic bladder aspiration. In certain circumstances, e.g. neonates, young children and females with repeatedly contaminated midstream urine specimens, the difficulty in obtaining a midstream urine specimen may be overcome by suprapubic blad-

der aspiration. This method has been used in a large number of neonates, children, pregnant and non-pregnant women with few complications. It should be remembered, however, that urine specimens obtained in this manner may have a lower bacterial count, e.g. 10^2 or 10^3.

The urine specimen should be rapidly transported to the laboratory, or if this is not possible, stored at 4 °C. Alternatively, it may be transported in a sterile container containing boric acid crystals which act as a preservative and prevent contaminants from multiplying. At the laboratory standard bacteriological procedures are performed. Two other methods of transportation and inoculation are:

1. The dip slide (Plate 1). In this test an agar-filled spoon or microscope slide with agar on one half is dipped into a midstream urine specimen and placed in a sterile container. Alternatively, the patient may urinate over the dip slide during the midpart of micturition. The slide is incubated for the appropriate time and there is a good correlation on quantitative bacteriology, comparing this method with standard loop methods.

2. Pad culture method. A dip stick consisting of a chemical reagent pad for the Griess nitrite test (see later) and a dehydrated culture medium pad containing colourless tetrazolium, which in the presence of bacterial growth produces discrete red spots, is dipped into the urine specimen. The density of the spots on the pad correlates with the number of bacteria in the urine specimen.

Types of Organism

The commonest organism in urinary tract infection is *Escherichia coli*, accounting for 80 to 90 per cent of all infections, and the incidence is higher in domiciliary practice (90 per cent) than hospital practice (60 per cent). The common serotypes found are 01, 02, 04, 06 and 75. Other organisms found in descending order of frequency are *Proteus mirabilis*, *Klebsiella*, *Staphylococcus aureus* or *Staph. albus*, *Streptococcus faecalis* and *Pseudomonas pyocyaneus*. The most common organism found in young boys with urinary tract infection, often associated with abnormalities of the urinary tract, is *Proteus mirabilis* (50 to 80 per cent). It is noticeable that these are the common organisms found in the faecal flora of normal subjects, and there is a close correlation between the organisms responsible for a urinary tract infection and the prevalent organisms in the stool in any individual.

The role of bacterial variants, such as protoplasts, spheroplasts and long forms (L), is of considerable interest and as yet ill understood. Studies in animals and man have shown that these forms survive in exceptional circumstances, e.g. high osmolality or in the presence of antibacterial agents, and then may revert back to their original bacterial form. It is interesting to speculate that the frequent relapse rate in urinary tract infection or the persistence of infection in renal tissue may be due to these variants.

Methods of Entry

It has been known for over a century that urine is an excellent culture medium; the urine of the female being better than that of the male and that of a pregnant female better still.

The Ascending Route

The vast majority of evidence indicates that in most urinary tract infections the ascending route is by far the most common method of entry. Several reasons have been proposed to explain the higher incidence of urinary tract infection in females.

The adult female urethra is approximately 5 cm long and has contaminants along the distal 4 cm. In infants faecal soiling and the close proximity of the perineum may allow further colonization of the urethra. Urethrovesical reflux, due to the negative pressure within the bladder at the end of micturition, allows some bacteria in the anterior urethra to enter the bladder. In adult life, urethral trauma during sexual intercourse is well described ('honeymoon cystitis'). Instrumentation of the lower urinary tract, at cystoscopy or by catheterization, is a well known forerunner of infection. There is a continuous column of urine from the bladder to the renal pelvis, thereby allowing any bladder bacteria to ascend into the renal pelvis and renal parenchyma if the defence mechanisms in the bladder are defective.

Haematogenous Route

For many years it was thought that infection carried by the blood-stream to the kidney was the commonest cause of parenchymal renal infection, but we now know this is not so. It is occasionally seen in severe septicaemia, especially with staphylococci, and is more common in children than in adults.

Lymphatic Spread

Although lymphatic spread can be shown in experimental animals, it is thought to be extremely rare in man.

Prostate and Paraurethral Glands

Chronic asymptomatic infection of either the prostate gland in man or paraurethral glands in women may act as possible sources for recurrent urinary tract infections.

Defence Mechanisms

It is well recognized that bacteriuria associated with frequency and dysuria often clears spontaneously without antibacterial therapy. Two possible mechanisms are responsible for this:

1. Hydrokinetic. This is a 'wash-out effect', where the total number of bacteria within the bladder is reduced during micturition. It is further decreased by the influx of fresh sterile urine from the kidney. Any significant residual urine left at the end of micturition will cause a defect in this defence mechanism.

2. Mucosal. The evidence for a mucosal defence mechanism came from studies which showed that if an inoculum of P^{32} labelled *E. coli* was applied to the exposed bladder of rabbits, only 0.3 per cent of the original inoculum was present after one hour. Although the radioactivity persisted, the bacteria had disappeared. This was not due to phagocytosis or the production of

antibodies. Likewise, secretory IgA, produced in human urine, does not appear to play a role. It is postulated that organic acids produced by the bladder mucosal cells have an antibacterial activity. In males, the low incidence of urinary tract infection has been attributed to the antibacterial properties of prostatic fluid. Finally, inhibition of bacterial growth may occur in urines with unusually low pH values.

Predisposing Factors

Age, Sex, and Race

The incidence of urinary tract infection increases with age, possibly due to the increased incidence of underlying abnormalities, such as bladder tumours, etc. The sex difference in incidence has already been discussed. Certain races, especially those with a high incidence of sickle cell disease or trait, are also known to have a higher incidence.

Hypertension

In large studies of females with urinary tract infection there is a small, but statistically significant, increase in blood pressure. It is not clear whether the hypertension predisposes to the development of urinary tract infection or vice versa.

Pregnancy

There are many conflicting studies on the incidence of urinary tract infection in pregnant women. Many early studies stated that the incidence was much higher than in non-pregnant women, and this could be attributed to three factors:

1. Hormonal dilatation of the ureters impeding urine flow.

2. Ureteric obstruction due to the enlarging uterus.

3. The favourable properties of urine from a pregnant female as a culture medium.

However, it is well known that 30 to 40 per cent of patients with urinary tract infection in pregnancy, if left untreated, will develop acute pyelonephritis. It has also been stated that there is an increased risk of toxaemia of pregnancy with infection of the urinary tract.

Diabetes Mellitus

From autopsy studies showing that the chronic pyelonephritis was common in diabetics and from poorly controlled clinical studies, it was thought that the incidence of urinary tract infection was increased in diabetes. However, more recent studies would not seem to justify that claim. Nevertheless, it is worth pointing out that a urinary tract infection, when it does occur in a diabetic, may predispose to diabetic coma and ketoacidosis, and management often involves catheterization. Urinary tract infection in diabetics is associated with papillary necrosis.

Instrumentation

Despite sterile techniques there is a four per cent incidence of urinary tract infection following catheterization of a normal bladder. This rises to 10 per cent in pregnant females and 30 per cent in patients with bladder neck obstruction.

Vesicoureteric Reflux

Vesicoureteric reflux is found in approximately 60 per cent of children with urinary tract infection occurring in the first six months of life and gradually decreasing to 10 per cent by the age of 10 to 14 years. Primary vesicoureteric reflux is caused by shortening of the submucosal segment of the ureter, due to lateral ectopia of the ureteric orifice. This defect is congenital in origin and, as there have been a number of families described where it has occurred in several siblings and in identical twins, it is thought to be an inherited defect.

Secondary vesicoureteric reflux occurs where there is some other underlying cause. It is stated that vesicoureteric reflux occurs as a direct result of urinary tract infection, a view that is fostered by the demonstration that reflux often disappears after treatment of the infection. However, in such cases it is highly likely there is some anatomical or innervation abnormality that cannot be demonstrated. The other causes of secondary vesico-ureteric reflux are bladder neck obstruction and the neurogenic bladder. Vesicoureteric reflux is graded:

1. Gross—pronounced dilation of the upper urinary tract during micturition.

2. Moderate—complete filling of the pelvicalyceal system without significant dilatation.

3. Minimal—incomplete filling of the collecting system without dilatation.

In gross vesicoureteric reflux, intrarenal reflux may occur leading to renal scarring, even in the absence of infection.

Obstruction to the Urinary Tract

Urine, which may be sterile initially, will become infected if left to stagnate, especially if catheterization or instrumentation occurs. Therefore any impedance to urine outflow, e.g. with congenital valves, neurogenic bladder, urethral strictures, tumour or stones, may lead to infection. Women with a residual urine volume of greater than 200 ml, 'the large bladder syndrome', are more prone to recurrent bacteriuria. However, obstruction occurring above bladder level is not usually associated with infection. From numerous animal studies it is known that obstruction within the urinary tract increases the susceptibility of the kidney to infection. The mechanism for this abnormality is not clear, but could possibly be related to increased tissue pressure, altered blood flow, or altered biochemistry of the renal parenchyma.

Miscellaneous Conditions

A variety of conditions predispose to urinary tract infection including hypokalaemia, various drugs such as analgesics and sulphonamides, and vascular disease or occlusion.

Susceptibility of the Renal Medulla to Infection

The renal medulla has a greater susceptibility to infection than the cortex, and from a variety of experimental animal studies certain facts have emerged. An inoculation of 100,000 organisms is necessary to produce infection in the renal cortex, compared with only 10 organisms in the medulla. The inflammatory response to such inoculation is delayed in the medulla. The high osmolality in the medullary region is known to interfere with the migration and function of polymorphonuclear leucocytes. Ammonia production, which occurs predominantly in this region, inactivates the fourth component of the complement system, thereby providing a more favourable condition for bacterial multiplication. Various bacterial forms, e.g. spheroplasts, protoplasts and L forms are known to survive better in the higher osmolality. However, the converse occurs with bacteria in the bladder as small numbers may persist and multiply during a water diuresis. The extrapolation of these observations to man is difficult, as conflicting results may be obtained using the same experimental protocol but using different animal species.

Pathology

The pathological changes in urinary tract infection depend on the site of the infection and its spread throughout the urinary tract. The presence of anatomical abnormalities within the urinary tract giving rise to obstruction, etc., will also change the pathological appearances. If the infection is confined purely to the bladder and urethra, inflammatory changes may occur, with polymorphonuclear leucocyte infiltration of the bladder wall. In severe cases, such as those associated with indwelling catheters, the inflammation may be intense with a haemorrhagic appearance.

The pathological changes occurring in acute pyelonephritis without obstructive lesions have not been fully studied, as this lesion is rarely fatal and therefore autopsy studies are extremely limited. Most information comes from renal biopsy, but again this is difficult to interpret because of the patchy nature of the lesion. In non-obstructive acute pyelonephritis the lesion tends to be wedge-shaped with its apex in the renal medulla and its base in the cortex (Plate 2). Histologically there are collections of polymorphonuclear leucocytes in the interstitium and occasionally in the tubular lumen (Plate 3). These may form microabscesses which destroy the renal parenchyma. Glomeruli are spared and survive as islands of normal tissue in the inflammatory mass. There may also be infiltration with chronic inflammatory cells, such as lymphocytes and plasma cells.

If the infection is associated with obstruction, the whole kidney will be involved and papillary necrosis may occur. Similarly, if the infection is part of the systemic infection, e.g. staphylococcal septicaemia, the whole kidney will be involved and the microabscesses will increase in size. The causative organisms may be cultured from the lesions, but are rarely seen on histological examination. In addition to the changes within the renal parenchyma there are inflammatory changes in the mucosa of the pelvicalyceal system. There is now a substantial body of evidence to suggest that so-called 'acute pyelitis', if it occurs, is an extremely rare phenomenon and the vast majority of patients with infection in the upper urinary tract have acute pyelonephritis.

Clinical Features

Urinary Tract Infection

Characteristically, the patient with urinary tract infection is female and between the age of 15 and 45 years. Abdominal pain may occur, initially suprapubic and often radiating into one or both loins. This gives rise to abdominal tenderness, anterior or posterior, especially in the line of the ureters. There is nausea and often troublesome vomiting. The patient is usually pyrexial and may complain of rigors. If there are no urinary symptoms at the time, the diagnosis may be confused with an acute abdomen, especially acute appendicitis if the pain and tenderness are right sided. Dysuria, frequency with the passage of small amounts of foul smelling urine and nocturia may occur. Haematuria, which varies from frank, even staining to the passage of small, old clots, sometimes occurs. Unfortunately the symptoms, including loin pain, do not help to localize the site of infection in either the lower or the upper urinary tract, although a significant pyrexia in excess of 38 °C is more common in patients with upper urinary tract infection. Although tenderness may occur in the loins, the presence of a mass may suggest the possibility of a renal carbuncle or a perinephric abscess.

In children the usual signs of urinary tract infection may be absent, but the diagnosis should be considered in those who fail to thrive or when there is the sudden onset of nocturnal enuresis in a child who is normally continent. Recurrent attacks of abdominal pain and vomiting in the absence of urinary symptoms may be a useful clue.

Asymptomatic bacteriuria has become increasingly recognized in hospitalized patients, especially the elderly with debilitating disease or those who have been catheterized. Patients with pre-existing renal disease may have positive MSUs. Occasionally, patients present with gram negative bacteraemic shock caused by overwhelming, but previously unrecognized, urinary tract infection.

The Urethral Syndrome

Approximately 50 per cent of patients with symptoms suggestive of a urinary tract infection do not have bacteriuria, and this has been termed the frequency dysuria syndrome or the urethral syndrome. It is commoner in females and often presents a problem in diagnosis and management. The possible causes are listed in Table 1.

Laboratory Diagnosis

Urine Analysis

Proteinuria may accompany urinary tract infection and will be 1 to 2+ on indicator sticks, but a quantitative 24-hour specimen rarely exceeds 1 g/24 hours. Small quantities of blood in the urine may be detected. In certain infections the urine is often alkaline because of ammonia produced by bacterial contamination, e.g. the urine is invariably pH 7 or above in Proteus infections.

Urine Microscopy

Microscopic examination, using a standard phase contrast micro-

Table 1. Aetiology of the urethral syndrome.

Infection		
Bacterial	—	Paraurethral glands
	—	Prostate gland
Protozoal	—	Trichomonas
Fungal	—	Candidiasis
Chlamydia		
Allergy		
Underwear		
Deodorants		
Soaps and bubble baths etc.		
Physical factors		
Sexual intercourse		
'Cold weather'		
Delay in micturition		
Hormonal		
Postmenopausal symptom		
Pregnancy		
Psychological		
Anxiety		

scope, of a freshly voided unstained centrifuged urinary sediment will help to confirm the diagnosis. If the bacterial count is more than 20 organisms per high powered field (Plate 4), it is highly probable that there will be significant culture of 10^6 organisms/ml. The commonest cells found during an active infection are white blood cells, representing an inflammatory response, but it must be stressed that infection may be present in the absence of cells. Likewise, these cells may be present in other renal conditions, e.g. acute glomerulonephritis in the active phase, phenacetin nephropathy and renal tuberculosis. The hallmark of the latter condition is sterile pyuria. The white cells in an active infection are numerous and characteristically present in clumps (Plate 5). Many reports have stated that it is necessary to have a certain number of cells present before making a diagnosis. However, this is not so.

If cells are absent from the urine but an active focus of inflammation within the kidney is suspected, it may be demonstrated using the prednisolone stress test. In this test the white cell excretion rate (normal below 100,000 cells/hour) should rise to greater than 200,000 cells/hour after an intravenous injection of 40 mg prednisolone. This test is useful in a patient who has already received a course of antibiotic therapy. The presence of white cell inclusion casts will confirm a diagnosis of acute pyelonephritis and help to distinguish it from lower urinary tract infection (Plate 6). In the past, the 'glitter cell', a leucocyte with specific staining characteristics with gentian violet and safranin, was said to be characteristic of acute pyelonephritis and not seen in lower urinary tract infections. The glitter cell has now been shown to be an artefact produced when white cells are suspended in a hypotonic solution. In addition to white cells, red blood cells may be present and the urine can be frankly haematuric.

Chemical Tests for Bacteriuria

Although the diagnosis of urinary tract infection depends on the quantitative culture of the urine, a number of chemical tests have been devised which may be useful adjuncts to screening procedures. The most-widely used tests are:

The Griess Test

The Griess test depends on the ability of bacteria to reduce nitrate in the urine to nitrite. The nitrite is then detected by a red colour change of a specific reagent. However, this simple test has the disadvantage of a high incidence of false negatives and certain bacteria, e.g. enterococci, do not reduce nitrate.

The TTC Test

In the TTC test bacteria at an alkaline pH will reduce colourless triphenyltetrazoliumchloride to an insoluble red compound. Four hours of incubation are required, and false positive results are found at pH values below 6.5 and with some strains of Pseudomonas, Proteus and Staphylococcus.

Blood Tests

In most cases of urinary tract infection a mild to moderate degree of leucocytosis is present. If the infection is uncomplicated, i.e. there is no underlying abnormality of the urinary tract, it is unusual for any degree of renal impairment to occur. Occasionally, some patients may have severe vomiting or circulatory collapse associated with Gram negative bacteraemia which will cause an elevation of blood urea and serum creatinine. If papillary necrosis occurs, renal function will be severely compromised.

Renal Concentrating Ability

A defect in the urinary concentrating ability with a reduction in maximal urine osmolality was first described in children with acute pyelonephritis. Since then further studies in adults with chronic and recurrent urinary tract infection and bacteriuric females have confirmed this defect. It has been postulated that either the presence of bacteria in the medulla may affect the concentrating mechanism or, alternatively, endotoxin produced locally could alter intrarenal blood flow or sodium transport.

Radiology

The role of radiological investigation in urinary tract infection is:

1. To establish a possible aetiology.

2. To determine the result of any damage caused by the infection.

3. To monitor the appearance of scars and growth of the kidney after the infection.

In adults it is unusual for radiological abnormalities to be detected during acute 'non-obstructive' pyelonephritis. The abnormalities which may occur are a decrease of contrast medium, together with some localized swelling and compression of one or more calyces. If the infection is complicated by papillary necrosis, the radiological function of the kidney will be decreased and it may be possible to see the so-called ring sign, if a papilla is loose in the renal pelvis.

   If infection has occurred during childhood, there may be renal scars which are areas of reduction and thickness of the renal cortex overlying a clubbed calyx (Figure 2). A renal scar with normal looking calyces indicates that the aetiology is not infection, but for example, vascular damage. Vesicoureteric reflux demonstrated by a micturating cystogram is less frequent in adults than children. Congenital abnormalities, such as duplication of the urinary tract, ectopic ureters and polycystic kidneys, may be found giving rise to infection. Obstruction occurs, either at the bladder neck level or higher, with dilated ureters and pelvicalyceal system. The 'large bladder syndrome' may be diagnosed on the postmicturitional film. Other abnormalities which predispose to infection are bladder tumours and calculi within the renal tract, i.e. kidneys, renal pelvis or bladder. If obstruction is found, then it is necessary to perform retrograde pyelography to determine the exact site of the obstruction and its aetiology.

Figure 2. *A renal scar overlying a dilated calyx in the upper pole of the right kidney.*

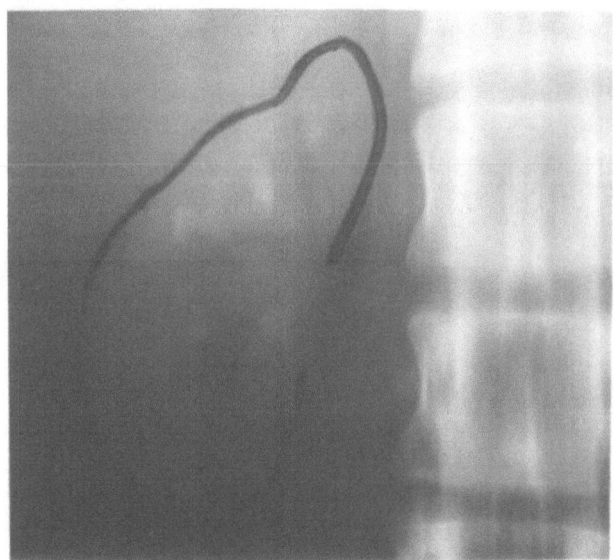

A higher incidence of radiological abnormalities is found in children with urinary tract infection. The most common of these is vesicoureteric reflux, found in 30 to 50 per cent of children with urinary tract infection, the difference depending on whether the children are symptomatic or asymptomatic and on their age. Renal scarring has been found in 12 to 20 per cent of children with urinary tract infection and up to 60 per cent of children with reflux are shown to have scars. In recent years, the entity of intrarenal reflux (calicotubular backflow) and its significance have been widely discussed. Intrarenal reflux is seen on a micturating cysto-gram when radiographic contrast passes out of the pelvicalyceal system and into the renal parenchyma (Figure 3). It is most commonly found in very young children with moderate or gross vesicoureteric reflux and usually occurs in the upper or lower poles of the kidneys, where it is associated with renal scarring.

Figure 3. *Vesicoureteric reflux with minimal intrarenal reflux in the upper pole of the right kidney.*

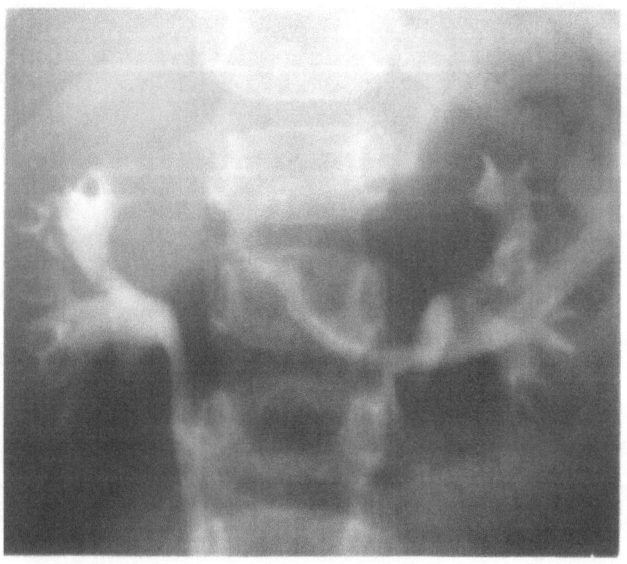

Who to Investigate and When

Opinions vary regarding the extent of investigations in patients presenting with urinary tract infection. As the detection of an underlying abnormality may be corrected and the infection appropriately treated to avoid deterioration in renal function, the following groups of patients should be investigated:

1. All children presenting with their first urinary tract infection or found to have asymptomatic bacteriuria.

2. Any infection occurring in a male.

3. A first infection occurring in a female, in association with haematuria, persistent proteinuria, sterile pyuria, impaired renal function or signs and symptoms suggestive of renal colic.

4. After two or more urinary infections in a female, even in the absence of the other symptoms and signs listed above.

Upper Versus Lower Urinary Tract Infection

When no radiological abnormalities have been demonstrated in a case of urinary infection, it is often difficult to determine whether the infection is confined to the upper or lower urinary tract. It is necessary to establish the site of infection, as this may affect the treatment and prognosis. As mentioned previously, the history and physical signs are often of little value. The presence of white cell casts, which are extremely helpful, may be absent in some cases of acute pyelonephritis. The role of the concentrating defect has not yet been fully evaluated, and renal biopsy, an invasive procedure, is often unhelpful.

Certain tests have been devised to elucidate the problem:

1. The Stamey Test. In this test bilateral ureteric catheterization is performed and urine collected from the catheters. If bacteria are cultured from the ureteric urine, this would indicate the presence of infection within the kidneys. However, this test is both time-consuming and inconvenient.

2. The Fairley Test. The Fairley Test is a simpler and less invasive test than the Stamey test. The patient is catheterized with a Foley

cathéter and the bladder drained. Fifty ml of 0.1 per cent neomycin sulphate is introduced into the bladder and left for one
hour. This is then removed by repeated washings using two litres
of sterile water, leaving the bladder empty. A specimen of the last
bladder wash is kept to ensure there is no antibacterial activity
remaining. Three further specimens are obtained at 10-minute
intervals and cultured quantitatively. These samples represent
ureteric urine coming from the kidney and bacterial counts as low
as 100 organisms/ml are significant.

In patients with upper urinary tract infection, elevated levels of
serum agglutination titres against the 0 antigen of infecting organisms have been reported in approximately one third of cases.
More recently it has been shown that antibody-coated bacteria are
found in the urine of patients with upper urinary tract infection,
but rarely in urine in lower urinary tract infection. The antibody-
coated bacteria are detected using a direct immunofluorescent
procedure.

Does Bacteriuria Cause Renal Failure?

For many years it was thought that the commonest cause of
chronic renal failure was chronic pyelonephritis. This view was
fostered by postmortem studies performed in the late 1940s showing that 50 to 60 per cent of patients dying with uraemia had
'chronic pyelonephritis' as their underlying histological lesion.
Some years later numerous studies revealed the increased incidence of bacteriuria in females, and the two facts were linked
suggesting that bacteriuria led to chronic pyelonephritis. Subsequently, doubt was cast on this theory.

The more frequent use of renal biopsy showed that in only one
third of patients diagnosed as having chronic pyelonephritis could
bacteria be demonstrated. Second, an increasing number of
pathological changes due to other causes were being recognized
which previously had been labelled 'chronic pyelonephritis'.
Third, over the last 10 to 15 years, data have accumulated

from dialysis and transplant registers, in which it is shown that the overall incidence of patients coming to end stage renal failure due to chronic pyelonephritis is considerably less than the incidence of bacteriuria in the community. Moreover, less than five per cent of patients presenting with end stage renal failure have uncomplicated, unobstructive chronic pyelonephritis.

There has been considerable discussion about the role of vesicoureteric reflux, intrarenal reflux and urinary tract infection in the aetiology of chronic pyelonephritis. Initially it was thought that vesicoureteric reflux alone did not produce renal scars and that the presence of infected urine was required. Conversely intrarenal reflux, due to an alteration in the shape of the papillae, was considered sufficient. Recently it has been suggested that intrarenal reflux and urinary infection are required to produce a scar, and that refluxing infected urine may alter the morphology of the papillae and allow intrarenal reflux to occur. Only further clinical studies will resolve this issue.

In long-term prospective studies of bacteriuria in both children and adults, few patients with chronic bacteriuria have proceeded to uraemia. In one series of over 1,000 patients with normal renal tracts, 30 per cent of whom had chronic bacteriuria, there were no cases of deteriorating renal function. It is accepted that urinary tract infection will cause a decrease in renal function in patients with pre-existing renal disease. Most recently, long-term studies in schoolgirls with bacteriuria have shown that no new scars occurred in patients with normal kidneys at the start of the study, irrespective of whether they had treatment or not. In conclusion, it would seem that, provided a patient has a normal renal tract, bacteriuria only very rarely causes terminal uraemia.

Treatment

The symptoms of urinary tract infection often resolve spontaneously after a few days. This may be enhanced by frequent micturition and a high fluid intake. However, it is important that in the treatment of urinary tract infection bacteria should be completely eliminated from the urine, and this requires antibiotic therapy. Ideally, two midstream urine specimens should be obtained before treatment is started, but often it is only possible to have one. The success rate for the treatment is high, about 80 per cent in domiciliary practice, although it is lower in hospital where the incidence of resistant bacteria is higher, and the bacterial flora somewhat different. After the initial course of treatment, it is necessary to follow up the patient for some months, as the recurrence rate is high.

There is still dispute as to whether it is more beneficial to have high tissue levels of antibiotic activity or high urinary concentrations. The antibiotics used are shown in Table 2. It is customary to give a full course of antibiotics for 14 days in patients with urinary tract infection. Recently in females with recurrent infections and a normal renal tract, a three-day course of antibiotic therapy has been shown to sterilize the urine, with a low recurrence rate. As the vast majority of such patients will not develop terminal renal failure, it may be a sensible and economic proposition to treat them with short courses of antibiotic, provided that repeat urine specimens are examined two and four weeks post-therapy.

In patients with renal impairment the dose of certain antibiotics, e.g. gentamicin, kanamycin, tobramycin, must be reduced according to the glomerular filtration rate (GFR) and body weight, to avoid serious side effects. Tetracyclines and nitrofurantoin are to be avoided altogether in renal failure; the former cause a decrease in renal function and the latter produces a peripheral neuropathy.

Special Situations

There are a number of special situations to be considered. In pregnancy when infection has occurred, treatment is mandatory because there is a high risk of acute pyelonephritis. If infection recurs, then long-term therapy should be considered, but care should be taken to choose a drug with no adverse effects on the fetus. The use of tetracyclines, etc., in these circumstances cannot be advocated. In females with the urethral syndrome any underlying non-renal condition should be treated accordingly. Thereafter, management becomes increasingly difficult. Some relief can

Table 2. Antibiotics used in the treatment of urinary tract infection.

Drug	Dose	Range	Side effects	Comments
Sulphonamides Sulphadimidine Sulphafurazole Sulphametrizole	1-2 g hourly oral " " " " " "	E. coli., Prot., Staph. " " " " " "		Useful in acute infection " " " "
Ampicillin	500 mg 6-8 hourly oral i.m. i.v.	E. coli, Prot., Strep.	Penicillin sensitivity	
Amoxycillin	250 mg 6 hourly oral i.m. i v.	As ampicillin	As ampicillin	
Co-trimoxazole	2 tabs 12 hourly oral	E. coli, Prot., Staph., Kleb., Strep.		Useful for 'nocturnal therapy'
Cephalosporin Cephalexin Cephradine	500 mg 6 hourly	E. coli, Kleb., Staph., Strep., Prot.	Few	
Flucloxacillin	250-500 mg 6 hourly, oral i.m. i.v.	As ampicillin		
Naladixic acid	1 g 6 hourly oral	E. coli, Prot., Kleb.	Photosensitivity	Safe in renal failure
Nitrofurantoin	100 mg 8 hourly oral	E. coli, Strep., Staph.	Nausea	Useful in nocturnal therapy Avoid in renal failure
Tetracycline	250 mg 6 hourly oral	E. coli, Kleb., Staph.		Avoid in renal failure and young children
Doxycycline	100 mg 6 hourly oral	As tetracycline		Can be used in renal failure
Carbenicillin	1-2 g 6 hourly i.m.	Useful for Pseud., Prot.	Penicillin sensitivity	Monitor dose in renal failure
Mecillinam	200-400 mg 6 hourly oral	E. coli, Kleb., Prot.	Few	High sodium content
Gentamicin	80 mg 8 hourly i.m.	Most G negative, esp. Pseud.	Ototoxic	Reduce dose in renal failure and monitor levels Beware when using frusemide
Tobramycin	1 mg/kg 8 hourly i.m.	As gentamicin	As gentamicin	As gentamicin
Kanamycin	500 mg 12 hourly i.m.	E. coli, Kleb., Staph., not Pseud.	Neuromuscular blockade	Reduce dose in renal failure and monitor levels

be obtained using pyridium (an anti-inflammatory agent) or diazepam. There is little or no evidence that urethral dilatation has any benefit in this syndrome.

In patients with chronic bacteriuria there is disagreement over whether long-term antibiotic therapy should be given, perhaps using cyclical drugs, or whether short term courses are best. In the latter case the antibiotic is chosen according to the sensitivity of the bacteria in the urine and the advantage is that the risk of producing resistant strains is reduced and careful checks are kept on the patient using frequent urine specimens. When given, long term side effects may be encountered with certain drugs and antibiotic efficacy on a long term basis, especially in children, is questionable.

In female patients with a large residual bladder volume, who are prone to recurrent infections, therapy with co-trimoxazole one tablet or nitrofurantoin 50 mg nightly has been shown to be beneficial. Similarly, if infection occurs following sexual intercourse, then one tablet per night may avert a recurrence of the infection.

Patients with neurogenic bladders present considerable difficulties, and the inability to micturate is often overcome by the use of an indwelling catheter. Intermittent catheterization is preferable, as it is less likely to produce infection, and catheter irrigation with neomycin solution or noxytiolin (Noxyflex) should be performed at regular intervals. Hexamine mandelate (Mandelamine), acidification of the urine and suppressive therapy, i.e. co-trimoxazole one tab. daily, are helpful in preventing infection. However, once infection is present, it is often with a resistant organism, e.g. *Proteus* or *Pseudomonas*.

Failure Rate

Although the recurrence rate of urinary tract infection is quite high, the initial failure rate is much lower, unless there is some abnormality of the urinary tract. Failure to eradicate the infection may be due to a variety of reasons. The wrong antibiotic may have been chosen if therapy is started before the result of the urine specimen is available. The development of resistant forms may occur, if previous courses of the same antibiotic have been given,

and likewise the development may occur of L forms or protoplasts, which revert back to the bacterial form on the cessation of
therapy. Finally, if there is persistent failure of therapy, further
investigation should be undertaken to determine whether there is
an underlying abnormality. After antibiotic therapy for urinary
tract infection, follow-up examination of the urine should be
performed at one month, six months and one year after treatment.

2. Chronic Pyelonephritis

What is Chronic Pyelonephritis?

Chronic pyelonephritis has been an overdiagnosed condition since its first description over 70 years ago. By definition, it is a chronic process of parenchymal renal destruction by bacteria leading to small, shrunken kidneys and end stage renal failure. The diagnosis and pathogenesis are easy if there is some demonstrable abnormality of the urinary tract giving rise to a history and bacteriological evidence of repeated attacks of urinary infection. A problem arises with patients who present with hypertension or proteinuria detected on routine examination and in whom an intravenous pyelogram reveals one or both kidneys to be small, shrunken or scarred and no abnormality in the urinary tract. The histological finding is an interstitial nephritis, similar to that found in patients with well documented chronic pyelonephritis due to urinary infection. Hence, different terms were used to describe these patients, e.g. chronic childhood pyelonephritis, chronic atrophic pyelonephritis and chronic non-obstructive pyelonephritis. In the past two decades an increasing number of conditions that give rise to interstitial nephritis have been recognized, and it is obvious that these were responsible for some of the cases in the past where no abnormality of the urinary tract could be demonstrated.

It has also been shown that chronic pyelonephritis found at autopsy, which varied from 6 to 33 per cent according to various authors, has slowly declined in the last two decades. Using strict criteria for the diagnosis, e.g. the gross macroscopic appearance of

the kidney with dilatation of the calyx and thinning of the overlying renal parenchyma, the incidence may well be less than one
per cent of routine autopsies.

In this chapter the term 'chronic pyelonephritis' will be used, as
defined above, and chronic interstitial nephritis will be defined
according to its aetiology.

Pathology

The characteristic gross appearance of chronic pyelonephritic
kidney is a small kidney, often weighing less than 100 g, with a
scarred surface (Plate 7). If the disease is bilateral, the two kidneys
are often a different shape and size. The renal capsule is difficult to
strip from the cortex and the kidney is hard and difficult to cut.
There is thickening of the renal pelvis and the changes of chronic
inflammation are often present. In some cases there are wedge-
shaped scars running from the medulla out to the cortex.

The classical histological appearance is that of an interstitial
nephritis (Plate 8). There are areas of interstitial infiltration with
lymphocytes and plasma cells giving rise to tubular atrophy and
fibrosis. In some areas there may be tubular dilatation due to
tubular obstruction, and the dilated tubules are filled with colloid
material giving a similar histological appearance to the thyroid
glands, hence the term thyroidization (Plate 9). Occasionally,
there may be foci of active and acute inflammation within these
areas. Between the areas of interstitial infiltration there may be
areas of normal renal tissue. The appearance of the glomeruli
varies considerably from being well preserved, or even 'hyper-
trophied' in the normal areas, to complete hyalinization of the
glomerulus in affected areas; this is due to longstanding tubular
obstruction. A common finding is periglomerulofibrosis (Plate
10). If the changes are severe and widespread, the appearance is
that of the end stage kidney (Plate 11). Vascular changes in the
kidney vary from minimal medial hyaline change and intimal
proliferation to thickened and fibrotic changes in small arterioles.
If hypertension is present, then the arterioles in the unaffected
areas may also show changes of hypertension.

Xanthogranulomatous Pyelonephritis

Xanthogranulomatous pyelonephritis occurs in children and adults, is more frequent in females than males, and presents with urinary infection, fever, loin pain, weight loss and lethargy. There is often a non-functioning kidney on the pyelogram, but the retrograde pyelogram and arteriogram frequently appear normal. The pathological changes are an enlarged kidney with perirenal fibrosis and adhesions, the calyces are dilated and there are yellow necrotic areas in the cortex. These areas are characteristically infiltrated with foam cells containing lipid material and calcification may occur.

Predisposing Factors

There are a number of predisposing factors which lead to recurrent or chronic bacterial infection and chronic pyelonephritis. These factors fall into two groups (Table 3):

1. Mechanical, in which there is interference with the drainage of

Table 3. Factors predisposing to the development of chronic pyelonephritis.

Mechanical

Obstruction to urinary tract
  Congenital
  Acquired
Vesicoureteric reflux
Disturbances of ureteric or bladder function, e.g. spina bifida, paraplegia
Renal calculi
Pre-existing renal disease
  Hypoplasia
  Dysplasia, e.g. polycystic kidneys
Renal ischaemia, e.g. renal artery obstruction, nephrosclerosis

Impaired host resistance

Paraproteinaemias, e.g. hypogammaglobulinaemia, myeloma
Neoplasms, e.g. lymphomas
Immunosuppressive therapy
Diabetes mellitus

urine or circumstances which favour the introduction of bacteria into the kidneys.

2. Situations of impaired host resistance, where the host's defence mechanisms allow the kidneys to become unduly susceptible to infection.

Obstruction to the urinary tract and vesicoureteric reflux have been dealt with in Chapter 1. Disturbances of ureteric or bladder function, e.g. neurogenic bladder, give rise to chronic pyelonephritis. In this situation there is incomplete bladder emptying, which allows bacteria to multiply. In addition the defence mechanism of micturition is absent. Vesicoureteric reflux also occurs with the development of megaureters or hydroureter.

Renal calculi and nephrocalcinosis may be the cause of chronic pyelonephritis in some cases, or, conversely, it has been suggested that chronic pyelonephritis predisposes to renal calculus formation (Plate 12). In the former situation, there is interference with urine drainage from the calyces or pelvis and intrarenal obstruction occurs. It has also been suggested that small plaques or groups of cells produced in an infection act as a nidus for calculus formation.

Other forms of pre-existing renal disease, especially where there is alteration of the normal architecture within the renal pelvis or parenchyma, may predispose to chronic infections, e.g. polycystic kidneys. In the management of any patient with pre-existing renal disease it is mandatory to take routine urine cultures and to treat the patients appropriately. Ischaemic kidneys also seem more prone to chronic pyelonephritis; this may occur with renal artery obstruction, and it is thought that the nephrosclerotic kidney of old age fits in this category.

Any condition in which there is impaired host resistance (e.g. hypogammaglobulinaemia and myeloma) makes the kidney more susceptible to infection. In myeloma, however, there is also structural damage to renal parenchyma. Similarly, with diabetes mellitus the role of host resistance has to be considered in addition to the development of diabetic glomerulosclerosis and the ischaemia produced by the vascular disease characteristic of the diabetic kidney. Patients receiving immunosuppressive therapy, for whatever cause, are more prone to infection; for example, the incidence of urinary infection is high in renal transplant recipients. However, in that case, there are also mechanical factors involved, i.e. altered drainage and structural damage due to homograft rejection.

Other Forms of Chronic Interstitial Nephritis

There are other non-bacterial causes of chronic interstitial nephritis. The recognition of these conditions has led to a greater understanding of the aetiology of 'small shrunken kidneys' and helps to explain why, despite the much higher incidence of urinary tract infection in females, the incidence of chronic pyelonephritis is roughly equal in both sexes. The various causes for this histological lesion are given in Table 4.

Congenital Causes

In medullary cystic disease (nephrophthisis) the characteristic changes of interstitial nephritis are seen in the medulla and the cortex, adjacent to the cystic areas, and progression of this lesion will lead ultimately to chronic renal failure. The renal manifestations of sickle cell disease are numerous, and interstitial nephritis, together with papillary necrosis, due to ischaemic vascular lesions within the renal papillae, may occur.

Mechanical Causes

Obstruction to the renal tract, especially high obstructing lesions, will give rise to the 'chronic atrophic pyelonephritis'. There is progressive destruction of renal tissue with tubular atrophy and interstitial inflammatory changes, produced by a combination of back pressure and ischaemia due to alteration of intrarenal blood flow. These changes may occur in the absence of infection.

The role of vesicoureteric reflux in interstitial nephritis was debated for many years, but the elegant experiments performed by Hodson and his colleagues (1975) have shed considerable light on the problem. Characteristically the changes associated with

Table 4. Non-bacterial causes of chronic interstitial nephritis.

Congenital

Medullary cystic disease
Sickle cell disease

Mechanical

Obstruction
Reflux

Metabolic

Potassium depletion
Hyperuricaemia
Nephrocalcinosis
Diabetes mellitus

Vascular

Hypertension
Radiation to the kidney
Ageing

Drugs and poisons

Analgesic abuse
Sulphonamides
Anticonvulsants
Lead poisoning

Miscellaneous

Balkan nephropathy
Acute tubular necrosis
Renal transplantation

reflux are found in childhood, and, if large scars in either pole of the kidney are seen in an adult, it must be assumed that these have been present since childhood. Initially it was thought that infection had to be present to produce such scars. However, it has been shown that reflux can occur not only into the renal pelvis, but also into the renal parenchyma. This is most likely at both upper and lower poles, and it is thought that the difference in the opening of the collecting ducts into the renal papillae in these areas makes them prone to develop the lesion. As our understanding of the aetiology of chronic pyelonephritis increases it may well be that chronic pyelonephritis becomes a term reserved for the end result of urinary tract infection and vesicoureteric reflux occurring in childhood.

Metabolic Causes

There are a number of metabolic conditions which lead to the development of interstitial nephritis. The glomerular lesions in diabetes mellitus are well known but such patients also have an increased incidence of interstitial lesions. These are attributed to the vascular changes that occur in diabetic kidneys.

Patients with longstanding gout are likely to develop interstitial nephritis due to uric acid deposition within the interstitium. The deposition of calcium will give rise to a similar histological picture. Potassium depletion leads initially to vacuolization of proximal tubules and subsequently to tubular atrophy and interstitial inflammation (Plate 13). This is seen in patients with potassium losing states, e.g. an excessive use of cathartic agents, diuretics, etc. It has also been shown that kidneys of potassium-depleted animals are more susceptible to infection, and therefore both acute and chronic pyelonephritis may compound the parenchymal damage already present.

Vascular Causes

Interstitial changes may occur as a result of damage to the intra-renal vasculature. This was seen in the past when the kidneys were irradiated in patients with intra-abdominal malignancy without adequate renal protection. However, the commonest form of interstitial nephritis due to vascular causes is seen in patients with hypertension, where the classical lesion of intimal proliferation and medial hypertrophy produces ischaemic damage. Elderly patients, who are known to have a modest reduction in overall renal size, also have an outer scarred appearance of the renal cortex. On further examination tubular atrophy and interstitial inflammation are seen in addition to the glomerulosclerosis.

Analgesic Nephropathy

Initially it was thought that the ingestion of analgesics increased the susceptibility to the development of pathological changes within the kidney. However, after extensive studies in many patients, in whom urinary tract infections had never been documented, it is now recognized that the analgesics themselves produce the changes. Much discussion has taken place as to which particular analgesic is responsible, and the consensus of opinion is that it is phenacetin probably in combination with other agents, e.g. aspirin and caffeine. Such compounds were easy to purchase without a prescription, and many patients with analgesic nephropathy have ingested many kilograms of these drugs over many years. In any patient with renal impairment a drug history must be obtained, asking specifically about analgesic abuse, especially in middle-aged females, or in any patient with a chronic painful condition, e.g. rheumatoid arthritis. The incidence of analgesic nephropathy varies from country to country and series to series. In Australia it is a major cause of chronic renal failure, and estimates in the UK indicate that it accounts for 12 per cent of cases of chronic renal failure.

In addition to the changes of interstitial nephritis (Plate 14), the other classical feature of analgesic nephropathy is papillary necrosis, where there is ischaemia of the papillae, which eventually become necrotic and slough into the renal pelvis (Plate 15). One should be alerted to this possibility if a patient with analgesic nephropathy presents with haematuria, a sudden decrease in renal function or renal colic. The radiological changes assist in making the diagnosis. The kidneys are small, shrunken and scarred (Figure 4), and if papillary necrosis is present, the 'ring sign' may be seen (Figure 5).

In addition to the renal lesion there may be peptic ulceration and an anaemia out of proportion to the decrease in renal function. Analgesic ingestion is often habit-forming, especially amongst females, and commonly there is evidence of excess barbiturate and alcohol intake as well. Renal function may stabilize or even improve, if patients can be persuaded to discontinue their habit.

Other Drugs and Poisons

Other agents capable of producing interstitial nephritis are certain

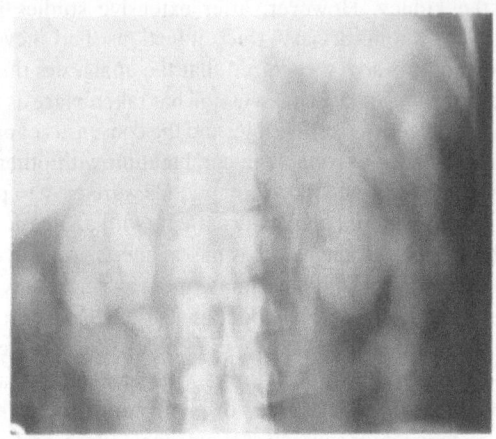

Figure 4. *Scarred kidneys due to analgesic nephropathy seen on nephrotomography.*

Figure 5. *The ring sign. A papilla loose in a calyx.*

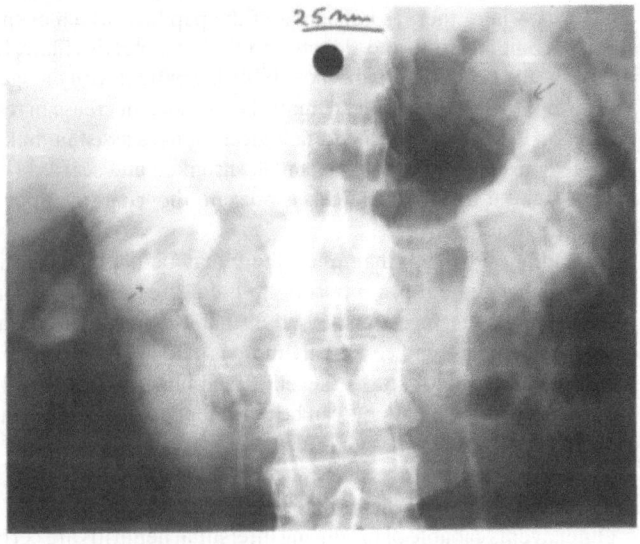

sulphonamides taken in large doses for a long period of time and various anticonvulsant agents. Poisoning, especially by heavy metals, may also be involved. Lead poisoning is the most common and is seen in people working in the lead industry or in those who have ingested quantities of lead from lead paint or plaster. There may be the other features of lead poisoning, such as anaemia, gastrointestinal and psychiatric disturbances. Patients who have lead poisoning and develop interstitial nephropathy often have attacks of gout, and hyperuricaemia is present which is out of keeping with the degree of renal failure.

Miscellaneous Causes

There are various immunological causes, the most notable of which is rejection of a renal transplant. Here, there is a vascular abnormality initially and subsequent progression leads to an intense inflammatory reaction within the interstitium. Following an episode of acute tubular necrosis, some histological features of interstitial nephritis may be found.

Another form of interstitial nephritis is Balkan nephropathy, which is not seen in the UK, but is endemic in Eastern Europe. In some villages this condition progresses to chronic renal failure in many people in the course of a decade. The aetiology is not understood, but could be due to some infective agent, possibly a yeast or fungus, occurring in the particular area.

Clinical Features of Chronic Pyelonephritis

General Features

Unlike oedema of the nephrotic syndrome or haematuria in acute glomerulonephritis, there is no hallmark of chronic pyelonephritis. Occasionally there is a history of recurrent urinary infections with dysuria, frequency and foul-smelling urine. Often there are no symptoms, and the condition is only discovered during the investigation of anaemia, hypertension and proteinuria found on routine examination. Such symptoms as lassitude, lethargy, unexplained abdominal pain or backache may lead the patient to seek medical advice. Occasionally the patient presents with some feature of chronic renal failure and is found to have end stage renal disease. Even then there may well be a paucity of symptoms, despite the virtual total ablation of renal function.

Special Features

Hypertension

The frequency of hypertension in patients with chronic pyelonephritis varies from 20 to 80 per cent, depending on the selection criteria used. The relationship between the two conditions is complex and as yet not fully elucidated. The question is which comes first—hypertension or pyelonephritis?

There are a number of facts to support the relationship. In women with urinary tract infection there is a small but significant increase in blood pressure over a comparable non-infected group. In addition, hypertension appears more commonly in patients with pyelonephritis than in suitable control subjects. In patients with pyelonephritis and hypertension, there is often a family history of hypertension, and hypertension tends to be more common in patients with non-obstructive chronic pyelonephritis than in those with obstructive lesions. It occurs in both unilateral and bilateral disease states. However, it is common for patients to have hypertension with normal or near-normal renal function, and the converse is also true.

Polyuria

One of the features of chronic pyelonephritis is polyuria. This may present as enuresis in childhood or nocturia, and only specific questioning will reveal this. Polyuria is a result of some abnormality of the countercurrent mechanism in the medulla which bears the brunt of the damage in chronic pyelonephritis. The failure of urinary concentration is usually out of proportion to the decrease in GFR. An alteration in the diurnal rhythm of electrolyte excretion also plays a role in the aetiology of nocturia.

Other Renal Tubular Dysfunctions

Failure of Acidification

The main contribution to urinary acidification occurs in the renal medulla, and lesions in this area interfere with the acidification mechanism. Hence, patients with chronic pyelonephritis may be acidotic with a low plasma bicarbonate and a raised plasma chloride level (hyperchloraemic acidosis). Some of the features of this syndrome are similar to classical or distal renal tubular acidosis in that potassium depletion can occur and there is increased urinary calcium loss. However, in contrast to renal tubular acidosis, patients with chronic pyelonephritis are able to lower their urinary pH values to below 5.5 provided the plasma bicarbonate is sufficiently low. As renal function deteriorates, the acidosis persists but the hyperchloraemia gradually disappears.

Failure to Conserve Sodium

In some patients there is a failure to conserve sodium and they present with circulatory collapse and hypotension. This defect may be seen in other forms of interstitial nephritis, especially analgesic nephropathy. The patients are hypotensive with an increased urinary sodium excretion in comparison to their sodium intake.

Chronic Pyelonephritis in Children

Unlike adults, where chronic pyelonephritis is often found as an incidental finding and is usually associated with a good prognosis (see later), the disease in children appears to take a more severe course.

The diagnosis should be suspected in any child who is failing to thrive or who has unexplained abdominal pains with nausea or vomiting. There is a tendency for such children to have severe hypertension which leads to chronic renal failure. If the course is prolonged and azotaemia is present, renal osteodystrophy will develop, resulting in stunting of growth and rachitic deformities (renal rickets). Occasionally fractures of the osteomalacic bones occur following apparently trivial injury. The growth of new bone in children is more susceptible to the factors responsible for renal osteodystrophy, especially the osteomalacic component. In such children, the 'renal tubular acidosis syndrome', with increased urinary losses of calcium, makes the failure of bone mineralization worse.

Investigations

The investigation of chronic pyelonephritis is twofold:

1. To establish the diagnosis.
2. To assess the degree of renal impairment and its consequences.

The hallmark of the diagnosis is finding infected urine, although it must be remembered that patients with other forms of paren-chymal renal disease have a high incidence of urinary infection. A positive midstream urine specimen should be found with organisms of the same type as found in acute urinary tract infections. In addition, examination of the urinary sediment will assist in estab-lishing the diagnosis. Casts, usually hyaline or granular, are often present. White cells and pus cells may be absent from the sediment or very sparse, and it is necessary to measure the hourly excretory rate of white cells before making a valid judgement. The rate is usually less than 200,000 cells/hour, but if the excretion rate is greater than 400,000 cells/hour, then the diagnosis of chronic pyelonephritis is highly likely.

Occasionally red blood cells are found in the urine and, the more active the disease process, the more informative the urinary sediment. Proteinuria will be found on simple testing but is usually less than 3 g/24 hours. The nephrotic syndrome, with a urinary protein excretion of greater than 5 g/24 hours, has been described but is unusual.

Impairment of the urinary concentrating ability may be estab-lished after a 12-hour fluid deprivation or by the use of pitressin tannate. Occasionally there may be high serum titres to the organism causing the urinary infection. However, the absence of appropriate titres does not exclude the diagnosis. Finally, if the diagnosis still remains in doubt, a renal biopsy may be performed. If an affected area is biopsied, the characteristic changes will be seen. However, from time to time areas of normal renal tissue are obtained from such patients!

Anaemia is present in chronic pyelonephritis, and it increases in severity as renal function deteriorates; this is usually normocytic and normochromic. If the disease is active with urinary tract infection, then a leucocytosis is to be expected. Occasionally some patients will have a decrease in serum potassium and most patients will have a period of hyperchloraemic acidosis. The degree of elevation of blood urea and serum creatinine will depend upon the extent of the renal failure. It is surprising that renal function often appears relatively well preserved in patients with radiologically small, scarred kidneys. Where there is radiological asymmetry between two kidneys, there is also asymmetry of renal function when determined by split renal function studies. This is most marked when there is moderate renal impairment and is especially true of the urinary concentrating defect.

Radiology

As with any renal disease a plain abdominal radiograph can give useful information. Reduction in the overall renal size is sometimes seen and mottled calcification, especially in the medulla, may give the first clue towards a diagnosis. The presence of renal calculi should be noted. The intravenous urogram, however, remains the main investigation from which the diagnosis is made. If the blood urea is raised or if there is poor definition with a routine intravenous urogram, an infusion urogram with tomograms should be performed. When there is gross focal scarring with obvious structural abnormalities in the urinary tract, there is little doubt.

In the absence of abnormalities one must rely on finding focal cortical scars overlying distorted or dilated calyces. These lesions may be unilateral (Figure 6) or bilateral. If only one kidney is affected, then its partner may be increased in size due to compensatory hypertrophy. In a case of unilateral kidney scarring, if the opposite kidney is not increased in size, it is most probably

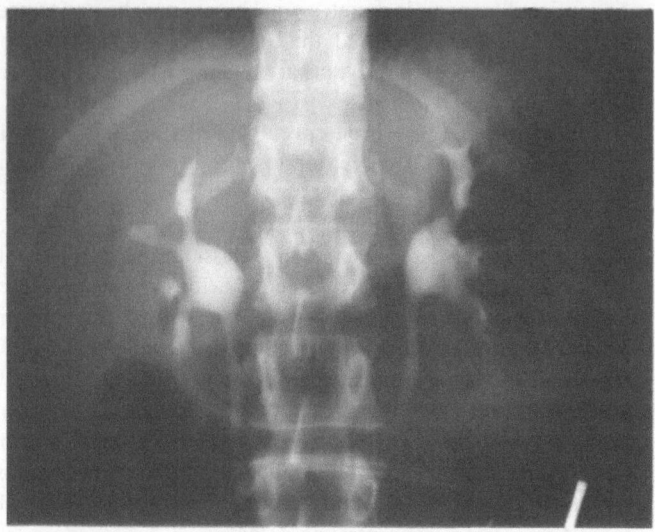

Figure 6. *Unilateral chronic pyelonephritis.*

affected, despite the absence of radiological signs. New scars will develop in children with vesicoureteric reflux if persistent or if recurrent bacteriuria occurs. The overall growth of the affected kidney is reduced by recurrent bacteriuria.

In adults, the changes described above are seen and it may be assumed that they have existed, albeit asymptomatically, since childhood. Occasionally, there is a grossly dilated calyx in an upper pole which stretches through to the renal cortex (Figure 7). However, more commonly the kidneys are small and shrunken with irregular outlines and a distorted calyceal pattern (Figure 8). This is in contradistinction to patients with chronic glomerulonephritis, in whom there may be a similar decrease in renal size but the outline is smooth and the calyceal pattern normal.

In the case of unilateral chronic pyelonephritis, the changes appear more commonly on the right. In any patient with marked

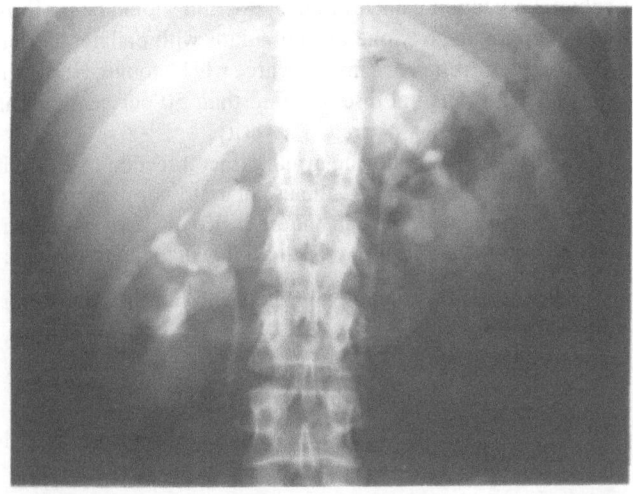

Figure 7. *Bilateral chronic pyelonephritis with gross calyceal dilation in the upper pole of the right kidney.*

Figure 8. *Bilateral chronic pyelonephritis.*

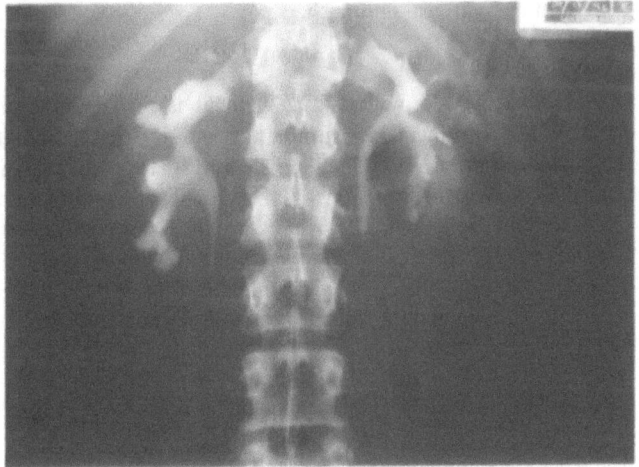

calyceal dilatation a micturating cystogram should be performed and in approximately one third of adults with unilateral disease, vesicoureteric reflux of a minor degree will be found. However, in patients with bilateral disease more than 50 per cent will have vesicoureteric reflux of greater severity.

The dangers of producing urinary tract infection or exacerbating existing infections make the use of cystoscopy and retrograde pyelography unnecessary in the majority of cases. However, it should be considered if any of the following situations exist:

1. Evidence of obstruction anywhere in the urinary tract on an intravenous urogram.

2. The finding of a non-functioning kidney with changes of chronic pyelonephritis on the opposite side.

3. In patients presenting with excessive haematuria or severe loin pain.

4. The suspicion of some other underlying pathology, e.g. bladder tumour, ureteric calculi.

Treatment

The management of chronic pyelonephritis requires a combined medical and surgical approach.

Medical Management

The initial part of medical management is the elimination of infection. The principles governing this and the use of antibiotics are similar to those described in Chapter 1. However, one must bear in mind that alterations in the dose of any antibiotic are required if renal impairment is present. Eradication of the infection can be extremely difficult in patients with anatomical abnormalities of the urinary tract or bladder dysfunction. Even in patients with no demonstrable abnormalities the failure rate is 10 to 15 per cent. Due to the pre-existing renal damage the rate of recurrence or reinfection is extremely high, with approximately 80 to 90 per cent of patients having a recurrence within 12 months.

After the elimination of the initial infection, attention must be

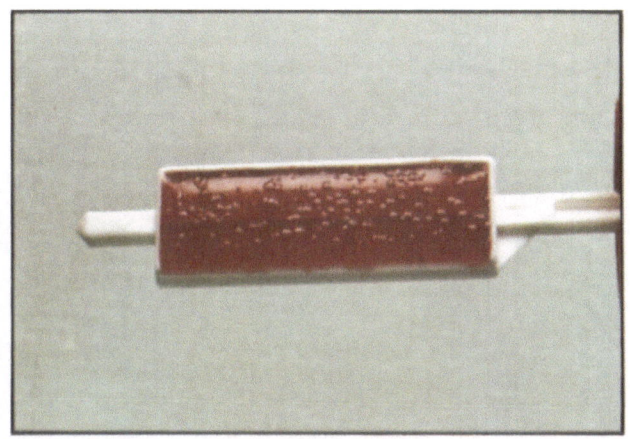

Plate 1. *A dip slide with numerous colonies of organisms.*

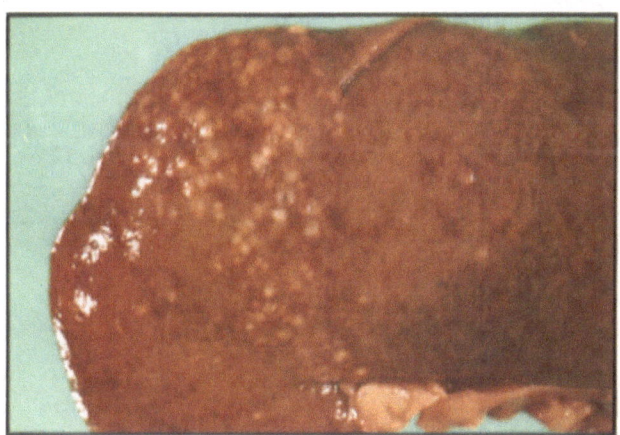

Plate 2. *Cortical abscess on the surface of a kidney with acute pyelonephritis.*

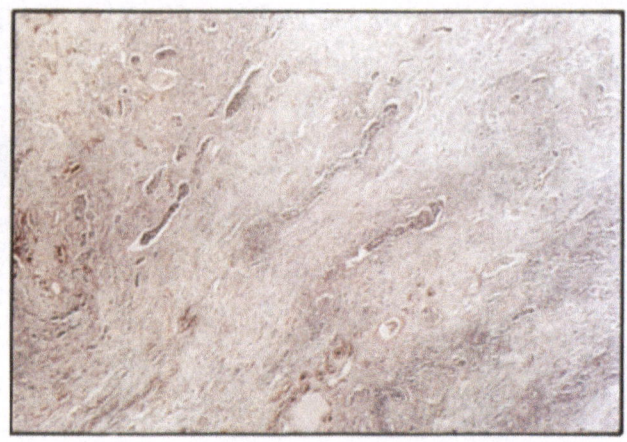

Plate 3. *Columns of inflammatory cells in the renal medulla in acute pyelonephritis.*

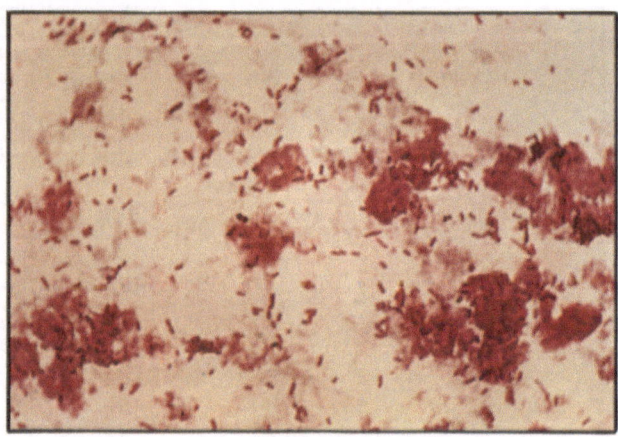

Plate 4. *Bacteria and white cell clumps in an infected urine (Gram stain).*

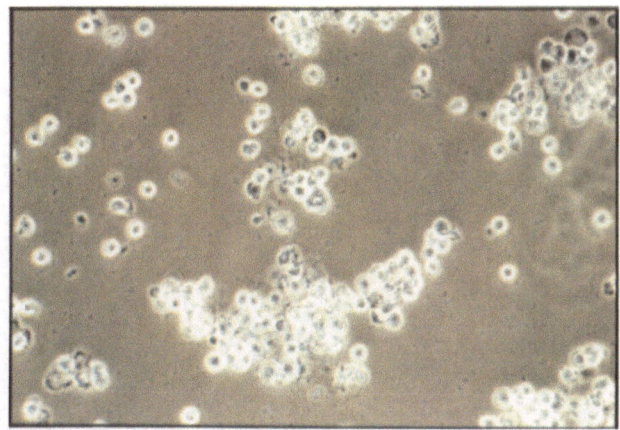

Plate 5. *White cell clumps in an infected urine (phase contrast microscopy).*

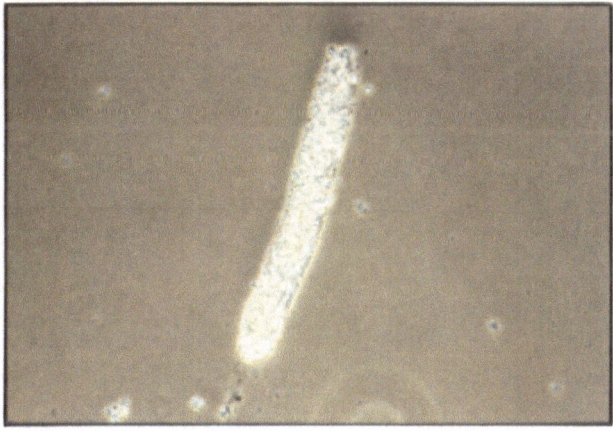

Plate 6. *A white cell inclusion cast seen in acute pyelonephritis (phase contrast microscopy).*

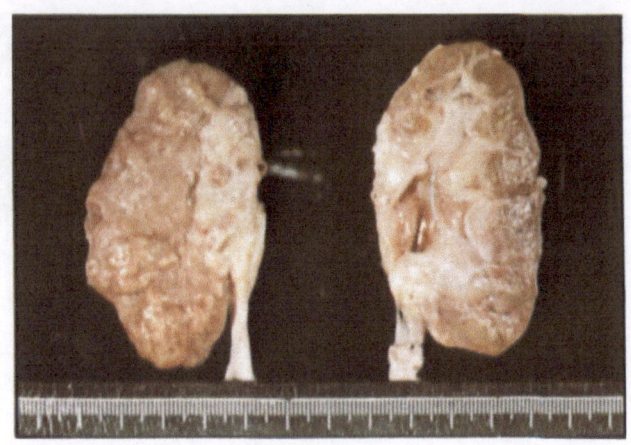

Plate 7. *Chronic pyelonephritis—small scarred kidneys.*

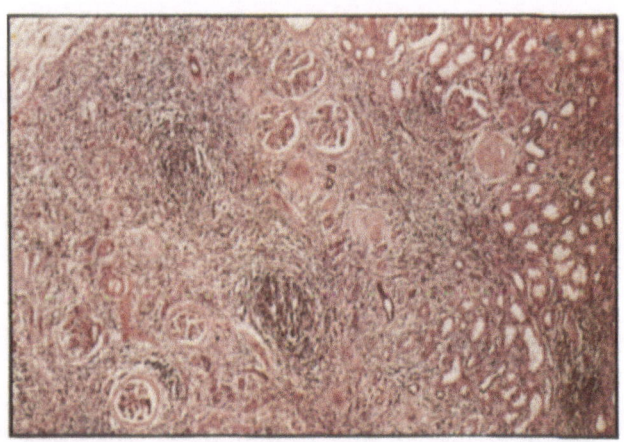

Plate 8. *Chronic pyelonephritis—histological appearance with interstitial fibrosis and adjacent normal appearance (H and E).*

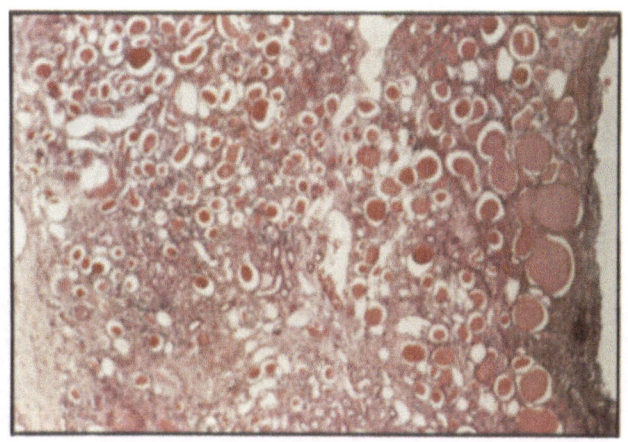

Plate 9. *'Thyroidization' in chronic pyelonephritis (H and E).*

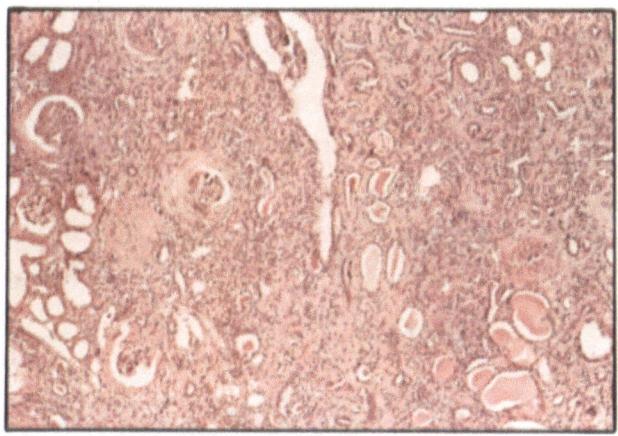

Plate 10. *Histological appearance of chronic pyelonephritis with hyalinized glomeruli and periglomerulofibrosis (H and E).*

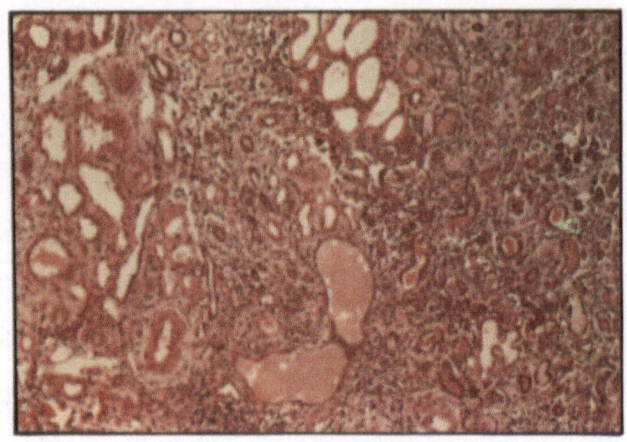

Plate 11. *The 'end stage kidney' due to chronic pyelonephritis (H and E).*

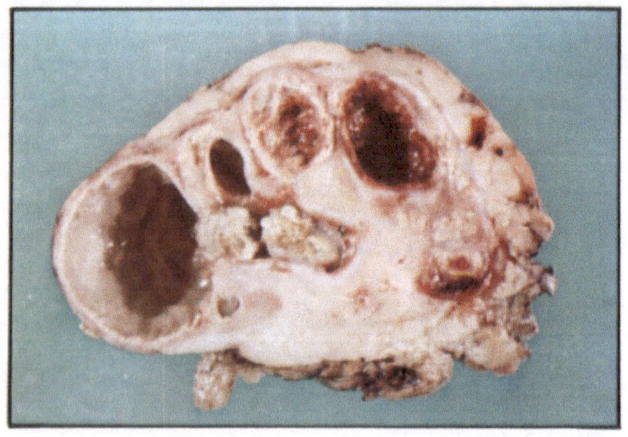

Plate 12. *Calculous pyelonephritis with a pyelonephrosis.*

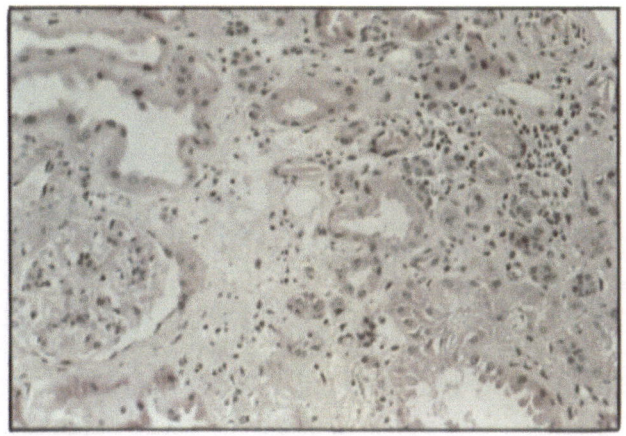

Plate 13. *Interstitial nephritis in potassium depletion with slight vacuolization in some tubules (H and E).*

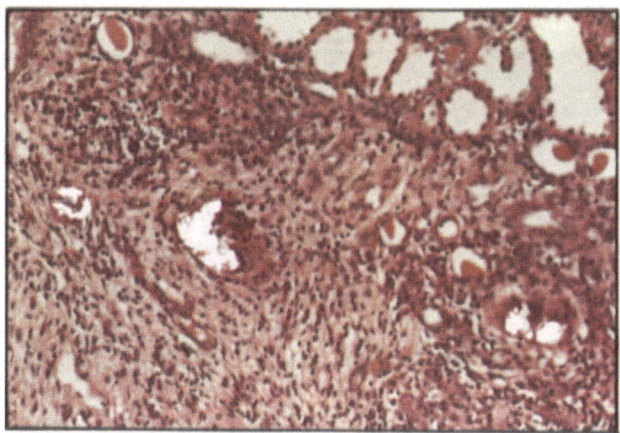

Plate 14. *Interstitial nephritis due to analgesic abuse. Also shown are oxalate crystals, an effect of long-term haemodialysis therapy (H and E, polarized).*

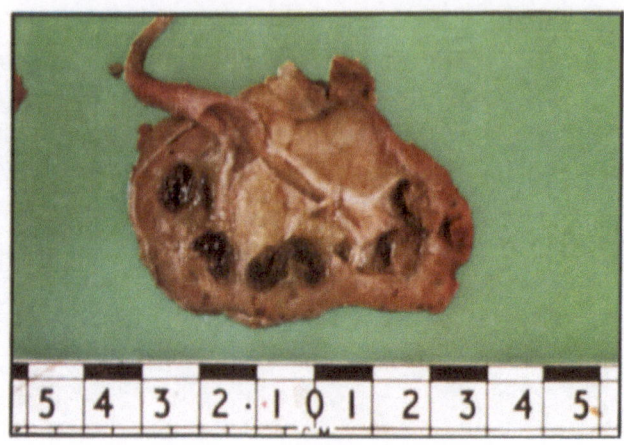

Plate 15. *Macroscopic appearance of papillary necrosis.*

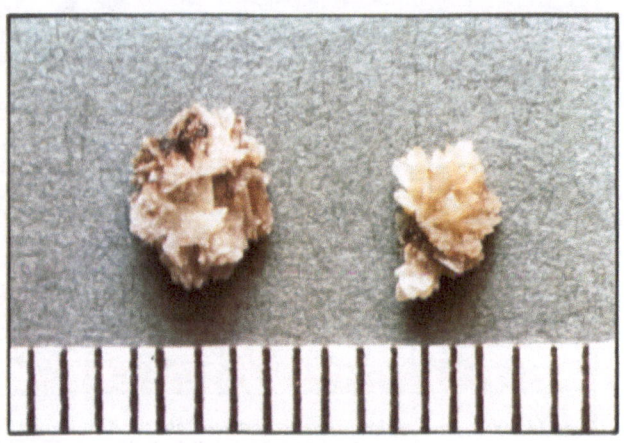

Plate 16. *Two calcium oxalate calculi (scale in mm).*

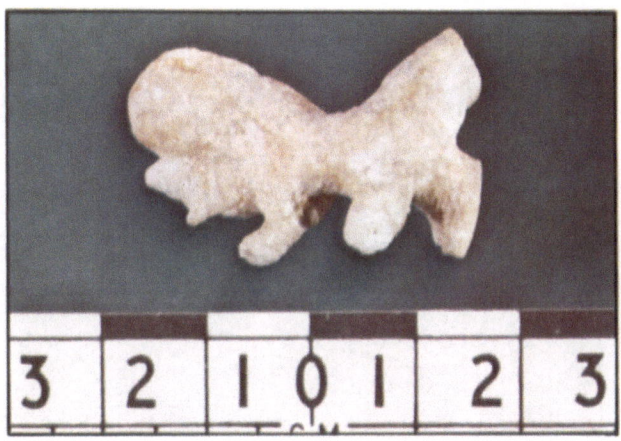

Plate 17. *Upper portion of a staghorn calculus (scale in mm). (See also Figure 10.)*

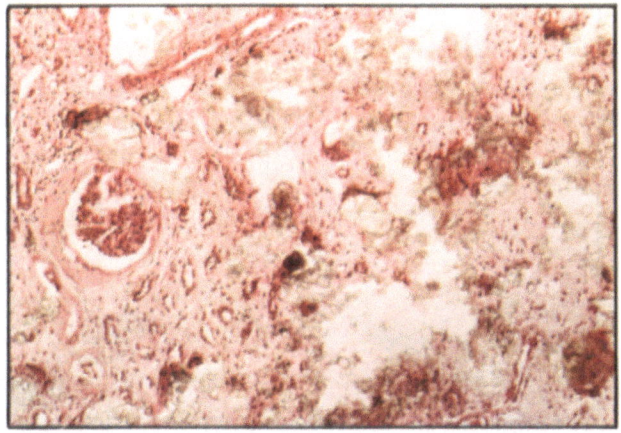

Plate 18. *Massive oxalate deposition in the kidney in primary hyperoxaluria (H and E).*

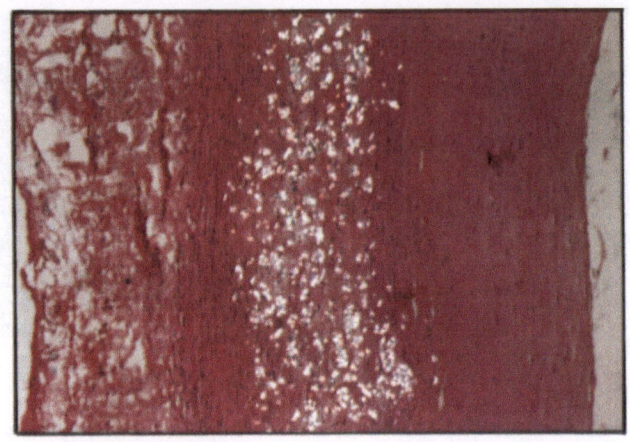

Plate 19. *Oxalosis affecting the aorta (H and E, polarized).*

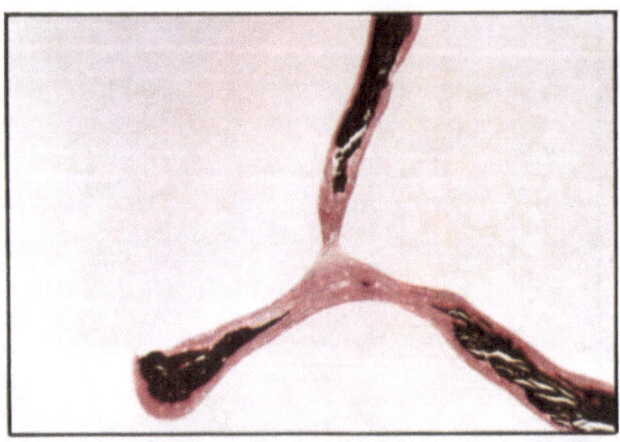

Plate 20. *Severe osteomalacia with wide osteoid seams on an iliac crest biopsy in familial hypophosphataemia. (See Figure 15.)*

paid to the prevention of any further renal damage, the most likely cause being reinfection. The management of such patients can be performed in two ways. The first involves regular, i.e. monthly, urine cultures and treatment given with the appropriate antibiotic. Second, continuous antibiotic therapy can be administered to suppress any infection. The danger in this latter course is that a resistant bacterial strain may be allowed to emerge during therapy.

However, in patients with chronic pyelonephritis who become pregnant and who have a urinary infection, the infection should be eliminated and the patient maintained on antibiotic therapy throughout the pregnancy. In this situation care must be taken to choose an antibiotic which is free of any side effects for the developing fetus.

Another cause of renal damage is the development and persistence of hypertension. Therefore it is mandatory that patients with chronic pyelonephritis have regular blood pressure recordings, and if hypertension occurs, it should be treated in the appropriate manner. Similarly, if the patient has an unrelated illness, the presence of chronic pyelonephritis and possible renal impairment should be considered when any drug therapy is given, to prevent further damage to already diseased kidneys.

Surgical Management

The role of surgical management in chronic pyelonephritis is the correction of any abnormality of the urinary tract. Hence correction of obstruction to allow free drainage, reimplantation of the ureter in gross vesicoureteric reflux and the removal of renal calculi are important.

If hypertension occurs in a patient with unilateral chronic pyelonephritis, the possibility of removal of the affected kidney should be considered in the attempt to cure the hypertension. The factors in favour of nephrectomy would be severe uncontrolled hypertension in a young person with elevated renal vein renin values and a normal contralateral kidney. In this situation, some would advocate renal biopsy of the 'normal kidney' to detect the presence of any disease or vascular abnormalities which might indicate that hypertension would continue after the nephrectomy, due to disease of that kidney.

Great care should be taken in managing patients with chronic pyelonephritis, especially those with a salt losing state, should they develop an unrelated illness or require any form of surgical intervention. It is essential that the patient should not become dehydrated and that extracellular fluid volume is maintained to prevent any further deterioration of renal function. Finally, when renal function deteriorates in patients with chronic pyelonephritis, they require management for chronic renal failure with dietary restriction, phosphate restriction, etc. until such time as it is necessary for the implementation of dialysis and/or renal transplantation. The details of such management are discussed in *Acute and Chronic Renal Failure* (Boulton-Jones 1980).

Prognosis

Recent studies have shown that uncomplicated chronic pyelonephritis has a good prognosis. In one large series of 200 patients followed for up to 11 years, the overall mortality rate was approximately 20 per cent. In another series, patients with unilateral pyelonephritis had an excellent prognosis, with 100 per cent survival over 10 years, and greater than 80 per cent survival at 10 years was recorded in patients with bilateral disease. The development of hypertension proved to be one of the factors responsible for the deterioration in renal function. Bacteriuria confined to the lower urinary tract did not appear to affect the prognosis adversely, although with upper urinary tract infection radiological damage was demonstrated. However, this was not accompanied by any changes in renal function and only further, more prolonged, studies will show whether this damage is of any significance.

In schoolgirls it is rather disappointing to note from recent results of treatment that new scar formation and the deterioration of growth of a kidney could not be prevented by treatment of bacteriuria in patients with abnormal urograms at the start of therapy. Conversely, it is encouraging that if the urogram was normal when treatment was begun, then no scars developed.

As a significant proportion of the patients with chronic pyelonephritis are females of child-bearing age, management of urinary tract infection and chronic pyelonephritis is important during pregnancy. Patients with chronic pyelonephritis are at an increased risk of developing pre-eclamptic toxaemia, especially if moderate renal impairment and/or hypertension are present. However, patients with radiological chronic pyelonephritis, with normal or only modest decreases in renal function who are normotensive can, with careful management, have a successful outcome to their pregnancy. In the absence of urinary infection, there is usually no further deterioration in renal function and some patients will have the usual physiological response of pregnancy, i.e. an increase in GFR with a proportional decrease in blood urea, etc.

3. Renal Calculi

Introduction

Calculi within the urinary tract are common and affect both adults and children. There have been changing patterns over the centuries and most early information indicates that bladder calculi were far more common in the past than now.

Incidence

Early information about urinary tract calculi was based on the incidence of bladder stones, and there have been several 'stone epidemics' in various parts of the world. In Norwich in the 18th century approximately one in 28 hospital admissions was due to bladder stones. In certain parts of Thailand, India and Turkey in the 1960s there were similar epidemics.

It is estimated that 2 to 3 per cent of all people in Western countries at some time suffer an episode of renal colic due to calculi. However, there is considerable variation, e.g. hospital admissions per 10,000 of the population are 1.9 in Sweden, 6.9 in the outer Hebrides and 9.5 for the USA in general, rising to 19.2 for the state of South Carolina ('the stone belt'). Less than one per cent of calculi occur in children, and there is a preponderance of males, especially with calcium stones, but the reverse is true in patients with so-called mixed or struvite stones.

Chemical Composition

The chemical composition of renal calculi varies widely according to age, race, socioeconomic status, country of origin and the presence or absence of urinary tract infection. There are two major components of all calculi. The smaller component, matrix, constitutes only 2.5 per cent of the dry weight of a stone and the remainder is composed of crystals. Approximately 90 per cent of all stones contain calcium. The common chemical constituents of renal calculi are: cystine 1 to 2 per cent, uric acid 2 to 5 per cent, apatite 15 per cent and magnesium ammonium phosphate with or without calcium (struvite) 10 per cent. The remainder are calcium oxalate, with or without phosphate (see Table 5).

Table 5. Chemical composition of renal calculi in Great Britain.

Calculi	Per cent
Calcium oxalate±phosphate	65–70
Calcium phosphate (apatite)	15
Magnesium ammonium phosphate (struvite)	10–15
Uric acid	2–5
Cystine	1–2
Others, e.g. xanthine	less than 1

In the matrix protein accounts for approximately 64 per cent; this is thought to be a small molecular weight protein (30,000 to 40,000) and is called 'matrix substance a'. Other constituents are sugars (10 per cent), glucosamine (5 per cent) and water (10 per cent), as well as citrates and carbon dioxide.

The structure of the calculi varies according to the crystals involved and their relationship to the matrix. Calcium oxalate calculi often have a small, rounded, clumped appearance (hemp seed, mulberry) or the 'jack stone' appearance with many projections from a central core. Some stones appear as small pieces of cinder or coke with a sharp, hard, sponge-like appearance (Plate 16). The struvite stone is characteristically a staghorn calculus (Plate 17) which, on section, has a columnar appearance. Uric acid stones tend to be smooth and rounded and have concentric growth rings with radial matrix striations.

Mechanisms of Stone Formation

It is generally assumed that crystal deposition occurs around a central nidus. Many theories have been proposed regarding the nature of the nidus. It is conceivable that cellular elements in the urine such as macrophages or bacteria, which are normally excreted in urine, act as a central focus. Plaques, occurring on the papillary epithelium (milk plaques or Randall's plaques), have also been considered, and there are stones which are attached to the renal papillae. There are also experimental data to suggest that there is maximal crystal concentration at the duct openings on the papillae, which gives rise to microstone formation. The microstone is in contact with urine in the renal pelvis which allows further growth to occur. The growth of the stone around the nidus is dependent on two factors.

Increased Concentration of Crystalloids in Urine

An increase in the concentration of crystalloids in urine may be produced in two ways:

1. Reduction in urine volume.
2. Increased excretion of the crystalloid concerned.

Mechanism 1 is known to occur in states of persistent dehydration. In troops transported from the UK to warmer, drier climates, the incidence of renal calculi increases significantly. Cultural habits regarding fluid intake are also important, e.g. the number of stone episodes was reduced from 0.85 per cent of the population per annum to 0.2 per cent in two comparable Israeli villages. In the latter case the villagers were encouraged to take additional fluids thereby increasing the daily urine volume.

Increased daily excretion of crystalloids is important in various metabolic states. This is true for calcium stones, but although 90 per cent of kidney stones contain calcium, two thirds of stone patients do not have an increased calcium excretion. However, oxalate stones occur as a result of a genetic condition, primary hyperoxaluria, uric acid stones in hyperuricaemia and cystine stones in cystinuria.

Physico-chemical Considerations

A number of physicochemical properties are important in the development of stones. These primarily affect solubility and the solubility product, i.e. the product of the concentrations of constituent ions in a solution. When the concentrations are below this product, the solution is undersaturated and if the concentration exceeds the solubility product, the solution is supersaturated. In this situation crystal precipitation may occur around a nidus of particulate matter or preformed crystals. Further increases in solute concentration lead to oversaturation.

In normal subjects a 24 hour urine is supersaturated with regard to calcium phosphate and calcium oxalate. The saturation is marginally greater in stone formers than in control subjects, due to a slightly raised urinary calcium in the former group. The increased urine calcium excretion leads to oversaturation and precipitation of calcium oxalate crystals. The urine pH is also increased compared to normals and this leads to oversaturation with the precipitation of calcium phosphate.

Urine pH

Alterations in urinary pH have a marked effect on the solubility of certain substances. The most florid example is uric acid, where the solubility increases many fold above a urine pH 6. Similarly, with cystine, solubility increases several times but the pH of the urine has to exceed pH 7 before the effect becomes marked. The reverse occurs in patients with struvite stones, where an increase in urine pH causes an increase in the magnesium–ammonium–phosphate products. As previously mentioned, an increase in urine pH is associated with increased precipitation of calcium phosphate, although the solubility of calcium oxalate does not appear to be pH dependent to any significant degree (Figure 9).

Matrix

The role of matrix in stone formation or growth is not clear. Occasionally large radiolucent matrix stones, composed primarily of mucoprotein with little mineralization, are found in the renal

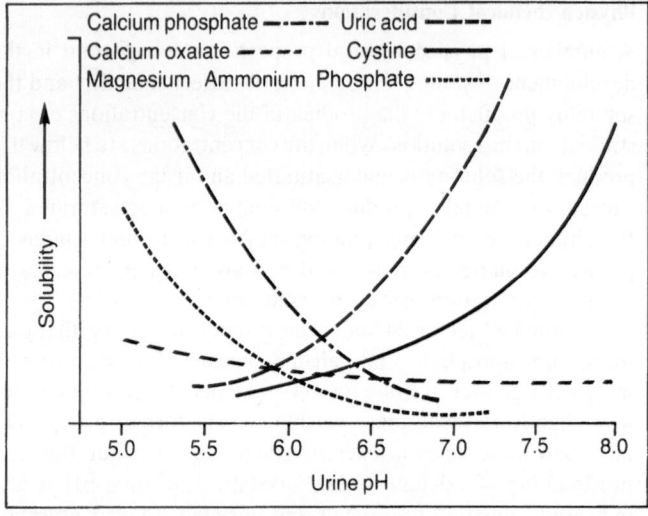

Figure 9. *The effect of pH on solubility of various urinary constituents.*

pelvis. It was originally thought that this mucoprotein influenced the growth of calculi by affecting crystal cohesiveness, and evidence was put forward to suggest that 'matrix substance a' was present in the urine of stone formers but not in that of normal subjects. More recently it has been suggested that the matrix acts as a non-specific coprecipitate, rather than as a promoting substance for calculi formation.

Stasis

Stasis within the urinary tract allows a longer time for crystallization to occur if the optimum conditions are present. Infection in static urine will lead to the formation of struvite stones if there is significant ammonia production from urea splitting organisms.

Promoters and Inhibitors

Certain crystals in solution can give rise to increased crystallization of other solutes, e.g. the presence of urate crystals may lead to increased precipitation of calcium oxalate, the so-called hyperuricosuric calcium oxalate nephrolithiasis.

The role of inhibitors of stone formation is complex. This mechanism must be important, as in normal subjects urine is supersaturated with calcium and other salts and therefore some form of inhibition must prevent stone formation. Experimentally, a variety of substances inhibit crystallization in urine, e.g. magnesium, citrate, zinc and fluoride, but their role in man is unknown. The earlier suggestion that there was a polypeptide inhibitor has been discarded.

Crystal precipitation and aggregation are inhibited by pyrophosphates, normally occurring substances which are excreted in urine. These substances affect a number of crystals, including calcium oxalate and calcium phosphate and some investigators have found that pyrophosphate excretion is decreased in stone formers. Pyrophosphate excretion can be markedly increased by the oral administration of orthophosphate, a substance used to treat recurrent calcium stone formers. The most powerful inhibitors of calcium oxalate precipitation are diphosphonates, but their therapeutic role is limited because of adverse effects on crystal formation and mineralization in bone. The mechanism of action of both pyrophosphate and diphosphonates is thought to be a delay in heterogeneous nucleation, crystal growth and crystal aggregation, possibly by binding to the crystal surface and thereby preventing further growth and aggregation.

Clinical Presentation

The classical symptom is an attack of renal colic, consisting of a sharp pain of varying intensity, starting in the loin, usually radiating into the groin and the testicle or labia and sometimes into the thigh. There is often repeated vomiting and anorexia and the patient may be pale and sweaty. Urinary frequency and haematuria may occur, especially if the stone passes into the urethra. The symptoms are usually relieved after the stone is passed, but the patient is often left with a sore, numb ache for 24 hours.

Other patients may complain of the passage of 'gravel' in the urine, with dysuria and haematuria. These symptoms may be mistaken for urinary tract infection. Occasionally patients present with persistent, dull, aching pain in one or both loins and are found on investigation to have calculi. In some cases there may also be a history of persistent urinary tract infections. Occasionally calculi may be symptomless and found on routine investigation for another unrelated complaint, or on further investigation for an incidental abnormal urinary finding (Figure 10).

Figure 10. *A symptomless staghorn calculus in the right kidney found during the investigation of microscopic haematuria in pregnancy.*

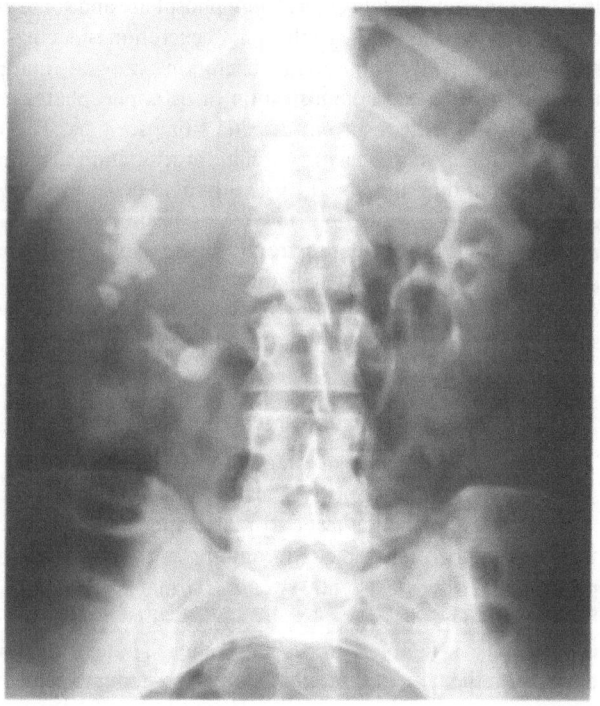

Investigations

Investigations are performed for two reasons:

1. To determine the aetiology of the stone formation.
2. To assess the degree of renal damage that may have occurred.

The 'work-up' of such patients is shown in Table 6. Hypercalcaemia and hypercalciuria are determined by serum and urine calcium estimations, the former being corrected for serum protein content. Hyperparathyroidism may be confirmed by an elevated serum parathyroid hormone level. Other metabolic abnormalities such as hyperuricaemia, renal tubular acidosis and cystinuria will be detected using such a scheme.

The radiological investigation includes a plain abdominal radiograph for detection of the stone initially, and at subsequent

Table 6. Laboratory investigation of renal calculi.

Serum

Fasting calcium, phosphate and alkaline phosphatase × 3
Renal function tests, e.g. electrolytes, urea, creatinine
Proteins
Uric acid
Parathyroid hormone

Urine

Microscopy and culture
pH (fasting)
24 hr calcium, phosphate, uric acid
Oxalate
Creatinine clearance
Cystine—nitroprusside test
　　　—amino acid chromatography

Radiology

Plain abdominal radiograph
Intravenous urogram
Micturating cystogram
Retrograde pyelography

Stone

Analysis

timed intervals to determine any growth or appearance of new stones. Intravenous urography should be carried out to determine the exact position of the stone and to assess any obstruction that might have occurred. It is highly desirable to obtain an intravenous urogram during an acute attack of renal colic as that is the optimum time to detect obstruction to the kidney (Figure 11).

Figure 11. *An intravenous pyelogram during an attack of renal colic. The right ureter and pelvicalyceal system is dilated.*

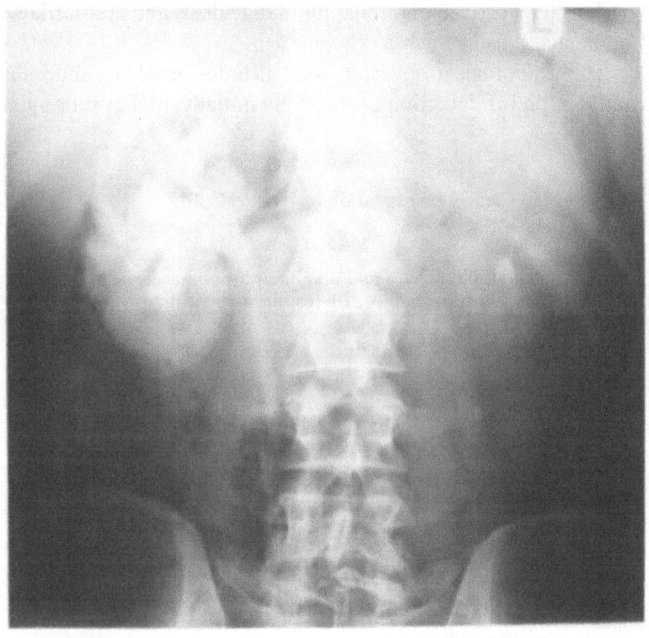

If a staghorn calculus is found in a young person, then a micturating cystogram is carried out to determine if vesicoureteric reflux is present. If obstruction at the pelviureteric brim or elsewhere in the ureter is strongly suspected, then retrograde pyelography should be performed.

Finally, stone analysis is extremely important if any calculi have been passed.

Types of Renal Calculi and Their Management

The various forms of calculi will be discussed according to the predominant chemical composition. Only medical therapy aimed at prevention or dissolution of existing calculi will be mentioned.

Calcium Stones

Calcium is found in 90 per cent of renal calculi and is the predominant element in approximately 70 per cent. The glomerular filtrate contains 9 to 10 g of calcium/24 hours and 98 per cent of this is reabsorbed in the renal tubule. The final excretion of calcium varies with a number of factors. There is a variation in urinary excretion with variations in the filtered load of calcium, and any decrease in filtered load due to a decrease in GFR, e.g. in renal failure, causes a decreased calcium excretion. Parathyroid hormone increases the tubular reabsorption of calcium and this explains why in primary hyperparathyroidism, when there is mild or moderate hypercalcaemia, calcium excretion may be normal.

Tubular reabsorption of calcium usually follows a pattern similar to that of sodium. Increases in dietary sodium will cause an increase in calcium excretion, and this may be relevant in certain areas of the world where the sodium intake is high and there is a high incidence of renal calculi. Similarly, the close link between sodium and calcium excretion may be used therapeutically. The effect of increasing calcium ingestion has a relatively small effect on calcium excretion. The ingestion of phosphate, however, decreases calcium excretion. Calcium excretion increases in metabolic acidosis because tubular calcium reabsorption is decreased. Fluctuations in plasma cortisone and thyroid hormone levels also affect calcium excretion.

The normal values for calcium excretion are up to 7.5 mmol/24 hours (300 mg/24 hours for males and 250 mg/24 hours for

females) in patients receiving a normal diet. Only one third of
stone patients have hypercalciuria, the major causes of which are
shown in Table 7, and an even smaller percentage have hypercalcaemia (fasting serum calcium greater than 2.6 mmol/1) (Table

Table 7. Major causes of hypercalciuria.

Dissolution of bone

Primary hyperparathyroidism
Immobilization
Carcinoma with bony metastases
Multiple myeloma
Osteoporosis
Renal tubular acidosis
Hyperadrenal states, e.g. Cushing's syndrome, steroid administration
Hyperthyroidism
Fanconi's syndrome

Increased absorption of calcium

Milk–alkali syndrome
Vitamin D intoxication
Sarcoidosis
Idiopathic hypercalciuria

Table 8. Major causes of hypercalcaemia.

Primary hyperparathyroidism

Neoplastic disorders, e.g. bony metastases, multiple myeloma

Sarcoidosis

Vitamin D intoxication

Milk–alkali syndrome

Cushing's syndrome

Hyperthyroidism

Immobilization

Idiopathic infantile hypercalcaemia

8). In large series of stone patients the proportion of underlying
diagnoses varies considerably, the commonest being idiopathic
hypercalciuria (6 to 40 per cent) followed by primary hyper-

parathyroidism, (6 to 18 per cent), with renal tubular acidosis and milk–alkali syndrome contributing less than 5 per cent. In 30 to 40 per cent of stone formers no obvious metabolic abnormality will be detected.

Hyperparathyroidism

Renal calculi and nephrocalcinosis occur in 60 to 80 per cent of cases of primary hyperparathyroidism, although it is unusual to have both in the same patient. Evidence of renal impairment is found in a high proportion of patients at presentation. This includes an elevated blood urea due to a decreased GFR and a defect in urinary concentrating ability out of proportion to the decrease in GFR. The latter, giving rise to polyuria, has been attributed to a defect in sodium transport in the loop of Henlé. The concentrating defect improves after surgical removal of the adenoma or parathyroid hyperplasia, following which there is a decrease in serum calcium but no change in GFR. Hypertension is common in patients with primary hyperparathyroidism and often persists when the serum calcium is normal postoperatively. Presumably this is due to parenchymal renal damage caused by nephrocalcinosis and/or superimposed chronic pyelonephritis.

The biochemical features of primary hyperparathyroidism are well known: an increased serum calcium with a decreased serum phosphate. However, this pattern is not always present and some patients may have a normal serum calcium, possibly due to vitamin D deficiency. Similarly, if the GFR is significantly decreased, then the serum phosphate will rise into or above the normal range. This presents a difficulty in distinguishing patients with primary hyperparathyroidism and renal impairment from those with secondary hyperparathyroidism due to chronic renal disease.

If bony involvement is present, the serum alkaline phosphatase will be raised and subperiosteal erosions may be seen on radiographs of the hands. The urinary calcium excretion may be elevated or normal due to increased tubular reabsorption.

Provocative tests have been advocated to distinguish primary hyperparathyroidism from the other causes of hypercalcaemia. In patients whose serum calcium is normal, phosphate deprivation will cause the serum calcium to rise. The cortisone suppression test may help to distinguish increased gastrointestinal calcium absorption, e.g. in sarcoidosis, from hyperparathyroidism. Oral prednisone reduces the serum calcium in sarcoidosis but usually has no effect in hyperparathyroidism. The diagnosis of hyperparathyroidism may be confirmed by finding an elevated plasma immunoreactive parathyroid hormone level either above the upper limit of normal or within the normal range yet inappropriate for the prevailing serum calcium level. The site of the adenoma can be detected by neck vein sampling.

Idiopathic Hypercalciuria

Idiopathic hypercalciuria is the commonest lesion found in any group of stone formers. It usually presents in the third and fourth decade, is commoner in males and a family history of renal calculi is often present. Hypercalciuria can be divided into two aetiological classes:

1. The commonest form is due to increased gastrointestinal calcium absorption giving rise to increased urinary excretion. Studies have shown that such patients have elevated levels of plasma 1, 25 dihydroxycholecalciferol, possibly reflecting the slightly reduced serum phosphate levels.

2. In a smaller group a renal calcium leak is postulated to account for the hypercalciuria. Initially it was attributed to an increase in parathyroid hormone, but this returns to normal when the urinary calcium is reduced by thiazides, so investigators concluded that there was a renal calcium leak and that the increased parathyroid hormone levels were due to secondary hyperparathyroidism. However, some patients in this group with a normal serum calcium and hypercalciuria have subsequently been found to have parathyroid adenomas on neck exploration (normocalcaemic hyperparathyroidism).

Other Conditions

Amongst the smaller group of calcium stone formers are a number of well recognized conditions. Renal tubular acidosis is dealt with in Chapter 4.

The milk–alkali syndrome, now rare, is usually found in males with a long history of peptic ulcer disease. The history of the ingestion of large quantities of milk which increases the calcium intake and large amounts of alkali which produces an alkaline urine (a favourable environment for the precipitation of calcium phosphate stones) should be sought in any male presenting with renal failure, hypercalcaemia, a normal alkaline phosphatase and nephrocalcinosis. Vitamin D intoxication rarely gives rise to renal calculi, but should be considered in any person who has been given vitamin D alone or in a proprietary compound vitamin tablet.

A syndrome of hyperuricosuric calcium oxalate stones has recently been recognized, where the stone is calcium oxalate but also contains uric acid. Hyperuricosuria has been found in these patients, usually males, who present in the fourth and fifth decades with calculi of unusual severity. Approximately 10 per cent of such patients also have idiopathic hypercalciuria. The underlying mechanism is thought to be increased nucleation and aggregation of calcium oxalate crystals caused by the increased urinary concentration of uric acid and urates. The hyperuricosuria may be a reflection of increased dietary purine content. Calcium stones are found in patients with medullary sponge kidney where there is stasis in the cystic dilatations of tubules in the renal medulla (Figure 12).

Treatment

It is essential when treating patients with calcium stones to find the underlying disorder. Treatment includes surgery for primary hyperparathyroidism, steroids in sarcoidosis and long-term alkalis in renal tubular acidosis. An increased fluid intake to reduce the urinary concentration of calcium oxalate, etc. should always be emphasized. In patients with calcium stones it seems logical that a reduction in dietary calcium is beneficial, and low calcium diets have been recommended. However, when the calcium intake is decreased, there is a significant increase in urinary oxalate excretion which predisposes to the calcium oxalate precipitation and, if

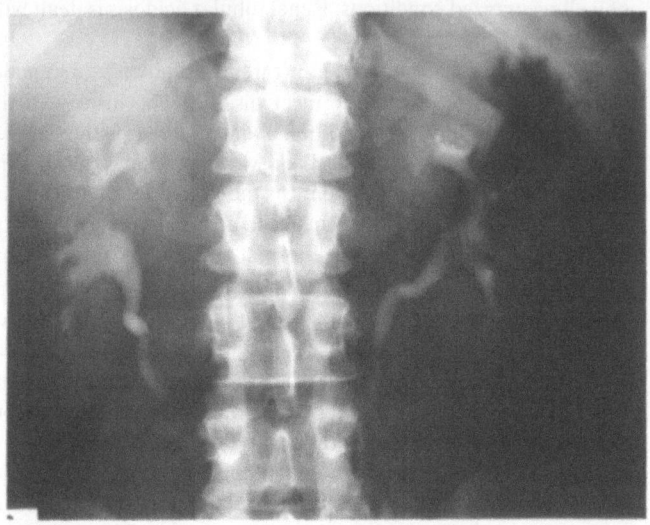

Figure 12. *Medullary sponge kidney with marked changes in the upper poles.*

such therapy is to be used, further dietary measures to reduce oxalate intake have to be employed.

A number of agents have been employed to reduce calcium excretion or to increase the excretion of inhibitory substances.

Thiazide therapy.   The use of thiazide diuretics has been claimed to reduce stone progression in over 90 per cent of patients. This effect is not seen with other diuretics, e.g. frusemide or spironolactone (frusemide increases urinary calcium excretion). The mechanism of action is not fully understood, but is thought to be associated with the natriuretic effect of the diuretic. With long-term administration, a degree of volume depletion occurs, resulting in increased sodium reabsorption. There is also an increase in urinary magnesium and zinc excretion, which are known to inhibit crystal formation and aggregation, and a decrease in urinary oxalate excretion. The most commonly used drug is hydrochlor-thiazide, starting at a dose of 25 mg daily, and increasing to 50 mg twice daily. Thirty to 35 per cent of patients have side effects including thirst, weakness and fatigue when starting therapy, but these problems can be overcome by reducing the dose or starting with a smaller dose. Other effects of long-term thiazide therapy, i.e. gout, diabetes mellitus and hypokalaemia, may occur and require treatment. It may be necessary to stop therapy in approximately 10 per cent of patients because of side effects.

Phosphate therapy. Various forms of phosphate are adminis-tered to patients with renal calculi for two reasons:

1. Giving phosphate will increase urinary phosphate excretion with a similar increase in inorganic pyrophosphates and these have a marked inhibitory effect on calculus formation. This approach is useful in both hypercalciuric and normocalciuric patients. It is necessary to give approximately 1,500 mg/day of elemental phosphate, which can be given as a variety of phosphate salts and proprietary brands, e.g. 'phosphate Sandoz'. Phosphate is contraindicated in patients with chronic renal failure and should not be used in patients with renal tubular acidosis or struvite stones. Phosphate has adverse effects on the gut and frequently causes diarrhoea. It can be especially troublesome in patients with peptic ulceration or the irritable colon syndrome. The use of sodium salts may cause fluid retention.

2. A different kind of phosphate agent, sodium cellulose phos-phate, is a resin which binds calcium in the gut. This limits calcium absorption and consequently reduces urinary calcium excretion. At the same time there is a decrease in urinary magnesium, but an increase in urinary phosphate. The resin is well tolerated and is given in a dose of 5 g, two or three times daily. It appears to be very effective in short-term studies but its long-term effects have not been fully evaluated.

Allopurinol. The use of allopurinol in patients with hyperuricosuric calcium oxalate calculi results in a marked reduction in stone formation. However, further long-term control studies are required before the full value of allopurinol is known.

Struvite Stones

The association between renal calculi, urinary tract infection and an alkaline urine has been known for nearly 80 years. Stones formed in such an environment have been termed infection stones, magnesium ammonium phosphate stones or triple phosphate stones. However, it is more common to use the term 'struvite' (magnesium ammonium phosphate) and such stones contain a mixture of this and carbonate apatite. The common staghorn calculi are frequently of this variety, as are the majority of bladder calculi. They occur in patients with spina bifida or spinal injuries giving rise to neurogenic bladders and in patients with ileal conduits.

Under normal physiological conditions an increasingly acid urine is associated with a rise in urinary ammonium. Certain bacteria possess the enzyme urease, which splits urea into ammonia and carbon dioxide causing a rise in the urine pH with the increased ammonia excretion. These bacteria include *Proteus*, staphylococci, *Klebsiella* and *Pseudomonas*; *E. coli* do not possess urease and are rarely associated with this syndrome. The alkalinity of the urine produces an increased concentration of the three components with an increase in the magnesium ammonium phosphate ion product and the presence of bacteria, cells and other debris in the urine provides a perfect nidus for calculus formation. It has been suggested that the presence of urease itself is important in the aetiology of these calculi and that its elimination may help the dissolution of the stones.

Treatment

Surgical removal of struvite stones is a necessary part of the treatment in an attempt to break the vicious circle of infected urine–calculi–further urinary infection. After removal of the calculi and correction of any anatomical abnormality in the urinary tract, it is essential to eradicate infection and maintain the urine sterile. More recently the use of urease inhibitors, such as acetohydroxamic acid, has been tried and although no dissolution of existing stones has been observed, there has not been a recurrence or progression of stone growth in short-term studies. However, the long-term safety of such agents has not yet been established. It is thought that struvite stones are associated with a high recurrence rate but a low mortality.

Oxalate Stones

Although calcium oxalate stones are extremely common, the vast majority of patients have no detectable abnormality of oxalate metabolism. However, in certain conditions urinary oxalate excretion is markedly increased and stone formation follows. Some urinary oxalate is derived from ingested and absorbed oxalate which is excreted unchanged. The majority comes from ascorbic acid, glycine and serine metabolism (Figure 13). Oxalate in solution forms highly insoluble calcium oxalate, whose solubility is unaffected by pH changes. Hyperoxaluria (normal 24 hour oxalate excretion 0.02 to 0.4 mmol/24 hours) is caused by increased ingestion and absorption of oxalate or oxalate precursors and increased oxalate production (see Table 9).

Figure 13. *Metabolic pathways of oxalate synthesis.*

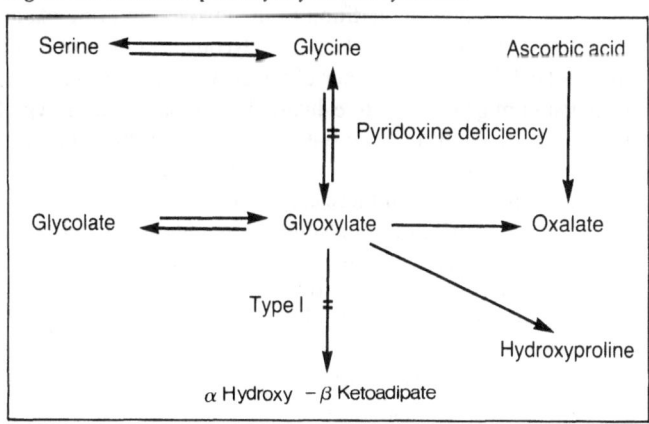

Table 9. Causes of hyperoxaluria.

Increased endogenous production of oxalate

Primary hyperoxaluria, type I and II
Pyridoxine deficiency

Increased ingestion or absorption of oxalate

Enteric hyperoxaluria
Foodstuffs, e.g. rhubarb

Increased ingestion of oxalate precursors

Ascorbic acid
Ethylene glycol ('antifreeze')
Methoxyflurane

Primary Hyperoxaluria

Primary hyperoxaluria is a genetic condition transmitted as auto-somal recessive, and presents with stone formation in early life. Death results from renal failure due to nephrolithiasis, neph-rocalcinosis and chronic pyelonephritis (Plate 18). As glomerular filtration decreases, so does urinary oxalate excretion, giving rise to oxalosis, where oxalate crystals are deposited in various tissues of the body, e.g. blood vessels (Plate 19), heart, bone, thyroid, pituitary gland etc. Two forms of this condition have so far been described. In type I, in addition to the increase in urine oxalate excretion, there is increased urinary glycolic acid excretion. The metabolic defect is a deficiency of the enzyme responsible for the conversion of glyoxalate, to α-hydroxy-β-ketoadipate. In type II primary hyperoxaluria there is an increased excretion of glyceric acid and the defect is probably in the metabolism of serine.

The treatment of both these conditions is a high fluid intake to promote a good urine output. Numerous agents have been tried to reduce oxalate excretion but with little success. Some patients present in later life and seem to have a better prognosis, but the majority die in early adult life from uraemia. Long-term haemodialysis and renal transplantation have been used in end stage oxalurics, but are associated with increasing extrarenal deposition of oxalate crystals.

Pyridoxine deficiency causes hyperoxaluria, but this is extremely rare, and the treatment is to give the appropriate vitamin supplement.

Enteric Hyperoxaluria

Oxalate stone formation is recognized in a number of bowel disorders and is due to the increased oxalate absorption from the gut. It is associated with malabsorption states, e.g. ileal resection, Crohn's disease and ileal bypass for obesity, etc. In this form of hyperoxaluria, glycolate and glycerate excretion are normal. Hyperabsorption of oxalate occurs and approaches 40 per cent of ingested oxalate, compared to only 12 per cent in normals. It appears to be related to fat malabsorption. The increased fatty acids present in the gut bind calcium salts and make less calcium available to bind to oxalate, which is then absorbed.

Treatment consists of adjusting the fat intake as well as medium chain triglycerides and, in some cases, increasing dietary calcium. Cholestyramine is effective in reducing urinary oxalate excretion and, wherever possible, surgery should be performed to reverse the malabsorption.

Increased absorption from increased ingestion of oxalate is rare, but occurs in various food fads, e.g. rhubarb. Increased ingestion of certain oxalate precursors gives rise to hyperoxaluria but usually the patient presents in acute renal failure. These precursors are ethylene glycol (anti-freeze), which is drunk by alcoholics, and methoxyflurane, an anaesthetic agent. The renal failure is due to oxalate deposition in the interstitium of the kidney and the treatment is the same as that for acute renal failure.

Uric Acid Calculi

Approximately 10 to 25 per cent of patients with primary gout and some with hyperuricaemia due to haematological proliferative disorders produce uric acid calculi.

There are three factors responsible for the development of uric acid stones. First, as with any calculus forming condition, a low urine output with a consequent increase in uric acid concentration will predispose to stone formation. This is especially true in hot climates, where the incidence of uric acid calculi is higher than in the rest of the world. Second is a high uric acid output from overproduction in gout or proliferative disorders. Third, and perhaps most important, is the solubility of uric acid in urine. Uric acid is relatively insoluble in an acid urine. There is a 20-fold increase in solubility in changing the solution from pH 5 to pH 7 (see Figure 9). It has been suggested that patients who form uric acid calculi have a lower urine pH than normals. Uric acid stones are usually radiolucent on radiographs.

Treatment

A high fluid intake, especially in the latter half of the day, is essential. Reduction of purine intake, e.g. in meat, is useful in patients with a high intake.

True alkalinization of the urine is often difficult to achieve but an attempt should be made to maintain the urine pH greater than 6.5 with the use of any alkali, the commonest being sodium bicarbonate. Considerable experience has been gained with the use of allopurinol, a xanthine oxidase inhibitor, which prevents the conversion of hypoxanthine to xanthine and xanthine to uric acid. Xanthine is a relatively soluble substance which can be excreted in the urine. The normal dose is 300 to 500 mg/24 hours. Occasional side effects such as skin rash, leucopenia and precipitation of acute gouty attacks may occur. The possibility of producing xanthine stones due to the increased urinary excretion of xanthine would appear to be theoretical as none has been reported so far.

Cystine Stones

Cystinuria is an uncommon inherited condition, in which failure of tubular reabsorption of certain dibasic amino acids gives rise to the formation of cystine stones. In addition to the excessive excretion of cystine, lysine, ornithine and arginine are also excreted. The failure of tubular reabsorption is due to a transport defect and a similar defect is found in the gut. However, this does not appear to have clinical consequences. The condition is inherited as autosomal recessive and the highest values of cystine excretion are found in homozygotes. There is increased excretion of cystine in heterozygotes, but it is rare for stone formation to occur in such individuals. Stone formation occurs in concentrated urines which are oversaturated, and especially at night. Like uric acid, the solubility of cystine is markedly affected by pH. The diagnosis of cystinuria is often helped by a family history of stone formation and by stone analysis. Cystine stones are radio-opaque due to double sulphur bonding in the molecule. A simple nitroprusside test is helpful in detecting cystine in the urine, which may be further identified by amino acid chromatography. Estimation of 24 hour urinary cystine excretion will help to distinguish the homozygote from the heterozygote.

Treatment

Treatment is aimed both at preventing stone formation and at dissolution of existing stones. It is important to increase fluid intake to maintain a dilute urine, especially overnight, and patients must be encouraged to drink a litre of water to produce nocturia at least once nightly. Alkalinization of the urine with sodium bicarbonate will increase the solubility of cystine. However, unlike uric acid stone formers, the urine pH must be greater than 7 and this is difficult to achieve. If these measures fail, the use of D penicillamine should be considered. This agent chelates cystine to form a soluble disulphide compound which is then excreted in the urine. The drug may be given in doses of up to 2 g/day, but it is necessary to check the urine carefully for protein as the side effects include the development of membranous glomerulonephritis. Some patients are also allergic and may develop leucopenia and a skin rash.

4. Renal Tubular Disorders

The function of the renal tubule is reabsorption of glomerular filtrate, which is accomplished with considerable efficiency; 98 to 99 per cent of all filtered water, sodium and bicarbonate are reabsorbed. Similarly filtered protein, glucose and amino acid are reabsorbed in order to preserve body stores. Reabsorption mainly occurs in the proximal tubule, but the final regulation occurs in the distal tubule.

There are a number of clinical syndromes in which the reabsorptive and secretory properties of the renal tubule are defective. As a result of this there are increased concentrations of normal urinary constituents and substances not normally found in the urine. The defects may be the loss of a single substance in the urine, e.g. glucose in renal glycosuria, or multiple substances, as in the Fanconi syndrome. Usually glomerular filtration is well preserved but it becomes impaired due to complications in the original defect, e.g. calculi in cystinuria and interstitial fibrosis in cystinosis.

The urinary abnormalities are caused by four mechanisms:

1. Acquired renal disease, e.g. chronic pyelonephritis or analgesic nephropathy giving rise to a sodium losing state.

2. Inborn or acquired errors of metabolism in which there is excessive production of a substance which is excreted in the urine, e.g. glucose in diabetes mellitus, and various disorders of amino acid metabolism, e.g. phenylketonuria (overflow aminoaciduria).

3. Inborn errors of metabolism giving rise to specific tubular defects, e.g. cystinuria, and renal tubular acidosis.

4. Inborn errors of metabolism where the tubular lesion is due to a generalized toxic effect, e.g. cystinosis, galactosaemia and Wilson's disease.

Conditions arising from mechanisms in the first two categories will not be discussed here.

There are a number of ways of classifying tubular disorders depending on whether the lesion produces a single or multiple defect and whether the lesion is in the proximal or distal tubule. The latter classification has been chosen (Table 10), but it should be remembered that a number of the defects affect both the proximal and distal tubule.

Proximal Tubular Disorders

Renal Glycosuria

As the filtered load of glucose rises, it is totally reabsorbed in the proximal tubule until the renal threshold is reached (10.1–11.2 mmol/l in normal subjects). Thereafter glucose is 'spilt' in the urine (see Figure 14). However, tubular reabsorption continues with increasing blood glucose levels until a tubular maximal reabsorptive capacity is reached (Tmg). In such a glucose titration study, as shown in Figure 14, Tmg is not a sharp cut-off point, but a small curve called the 'splay' and this is considered to be due to the heterogeneity of the nephron population.

Renal glycosuria occurs in two forms. The less common variety is found in the Fanconi syndrome, etc., where Tmg is markedly reduced. However, in the commoner variety Tmg is normal, but there is an increase in the splay and glucose is excreted in the urine below the normal renal threshold (Figure 14). This is due to decreased glucose reabsorption in some or all of the tubules. This should not be confused with the glycosuria that occurs in diabetes mellitus in which Tmg, renal threshold and splay are normal unless diabetic renal involvement has occurred.

The frequency of renal glycosuria varies between 0.1 and 2.0 per cent of the population according to the diagnostic criteria

Table 10. Classification of tubular disorders.

Proximal tubule

Congenital
    Primary defect of tubular transport
        Renal glycosuria
        Cystinuria
        Hartnup disease
        Xanthinuria
        Vitamin D resistant rickets (familial hypophosphataemia)
        Pseudohypoparathyroidism
    Secondary effect of extrarenal metabolic defects
        Cystinosis (Lignac–Fanconi Syndrome)
        Galactosaemia
        Wilson's disease (Hepatolenticular degeneration)
        Lowe's syndrome (Cerebro-oculo-renal dystrophy)

Acquired
    Adult Fanconi syndrome
    Drugs
    Heavy metals
    Multiple myeloma
    Nephrotic syndrome
    Amyloidosis
    Hyperglobulinaemia
    Idiopathic hypercalciuria

Distal tubule

Congenital
    Renal tubular acidosis
    Nephrogenic diabetes insipidus

Acquired
    Hypercalcaemia
    Hypokalaemia
    Lithium intoxication

---

used. It is inherited as Mendelian dominant. In the majority of cases the lesion is harmless if correctly diagnosed. Some diagnostic confusion may occur if glycosuria is first detected in pregnancy. The diagnosis is made by finding glycosuria with a normal fasting blood glucose level or in a non-diabetic glucose tolerance test. The other urinary abnormality which occurs is excess glycine excretion. As stated previously most patients are asymptomatic, but if

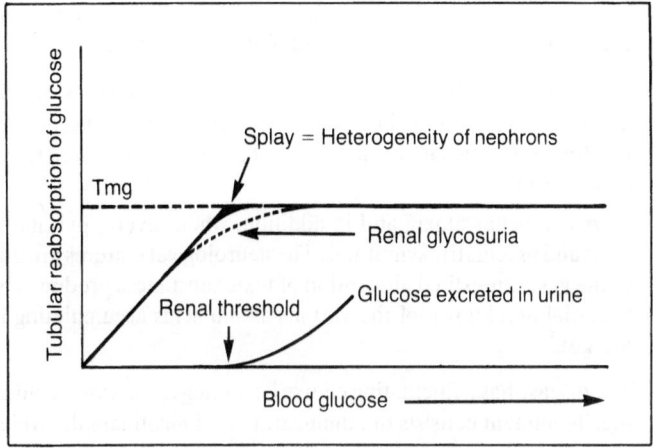

Figure 14. *Kinetics of glucose reabsorption in normal subjects and in renal glycosuria.*

the lesion is severe, it gives rise to polyuria and polydipsia, and extremely severe cases have been reported where ketosis has occurred. No treatment is required for the vast majority of patients unless ketosis occurs and then it is necessary to give increased oral glucose loads.

Cystinuria

Cystinuria is considered in Chapter 3.

Hartnup Disease

Hartnup disease is a rare disorder of amino acid transport with defects in both the renal tubule and jejunal mucosa. There are multiple amino acid losses in the urine without other defects, e.g. bicarbonate, phosphate or glucose. The amino acids excreted are those of the monoamino/monocarboxylic group, i.e. serine, glutamine, histidine, phenylalanine, tyrosine and tryptophan. The condition is inherited as an autosomal recessive and there is an increased incidence in consanguineous unions. Patients are usually below average height and have two symptoms:

1. A pellagra rash which is red and scaly in exposed areas, having a clear demarcation line. This is due to the absence of nicotinamide, caused by a deficiency of tryptophan required for its metabolism.

2. A cerebellar ataxia and in addition, when severe, pyramidal signs and psychiatric symptoms. The neurological features are due to the gastrointestinal absorption of toxic substances produced by bacterial breakdown of the various amino acids accumulating in the gut.

The disease has a fluctuating course becoming less serious in adult life. Treatment consists of administration of nicotinamide, which clears the skin rash, and a good dietary protein intake to improve growth. During cerebellar attacks an hepatic coma regimen, i.e. intravenous glucose and oral neomycin, should be used.

Xanthinuria

Xanthinuria is an extremely rare condition caused by the absence of the enzyme xanthine oxidase which converts xanthine to hypoxanthine and hypoxanthine to uric acid. Patients present with radiolucent stones and have an extremely low plasma uric acid and a high urinary xanthine excretion, this being accentuated by a tubular defect of xanthine reabsorption. Treatment consists of a high fluid intake and alkalinization of the urine, as xanthine is more soluble in an alkaline urine.

Vitamin D Resistant Rickets
(Familial Hypophosphataemia)

Phosphate is reabsorbed in the proximal tubule and undergoes similar reabsorptive kinetics to glucose, namely there is a tubular maximum reabsorptive capacity (Tmp). The renal phosphate clearance is controlled by several factors, including parathyroid hormone (PTH) which increases phosphate clearance. In hypoparathyroidism there is a decrease in phosphate clearance with an associated rise in plasma phosphate. The reverse occurs in hyperparathyroidism, i.e. phosphate clearance increases with a decrease in plasma phosphate.

Vitamin D resistant rickets is an inherited defect of phosphate reabsorption. The lesion is X-linked dominant with males more severely affected than females. It presents in infancy when the child has difficulty in walking, and the bony features—dwarfism, genu valgum or genu varum—appear. There is muscular weakness and the classical radiographic features of rickets. Tetany rarely occurs. When the disease occurs in females it is often milder and presents in later life with clinical, radiological and histological features of osteomalacia (Figure 15, Plate 20). The biochemical hallmark is the reduced plasma phosphate which is greater in homozygote males than in heterozygote females. Alkaline phosphatase is raised in the early years, but may be normal later. Plasma calcium levels are often normal or slightly reduced. Urinary phosphate excretion is markedly increased despite the low plasma phosphate. Faecal calcium excretion is increased, indicating a gastrointestinal defect in calcium absorption.

The mechanism of this lesion is not fully determined, but there are two possibilities. First, there is decreased phosphate reabsorption, i.e. Tmp is reduced due to an enzyme defect in the proximal tubule. Second, phosphate clearance is increased due to excessive PTH activity on the tubule, the excess PTH activity compensating for the impaired gastrointestinal calcium absorption. There is accumulating evidence to favour the latter explanation as an intravenous calcium infusion lowers the circulating PTH level with decreased phosphate clearance and decreased phosphate excretion.

Treatment involves giving large doses of vitamin D, 100,000 to 600,000 units daily. Plasma calcium levels should be monitored regularly to detect hypercalcaemia. In addition, it is necessary to give phosphate salts 0.5 to 1.5 g of phosphate daily. It is often difficult to increase the plasma phosphate, as large doses of phosphate produce gastrointestinal disturbances, e.g. diarrhoea and nausea. Recently, evidence has been produced to suggest that the vitamin D analogue 1, α-hydroxycholecalciferol is effective in increasing both calcium and phosphate absorption in these patients with healing of the osteomalacia.

Figure 15. *Familial hypophosphataemia. Right leg showing Looser's zones. (a) In 1942. (b) In 1978.*

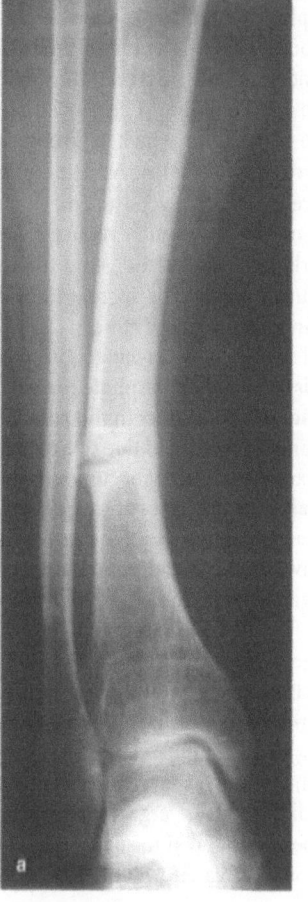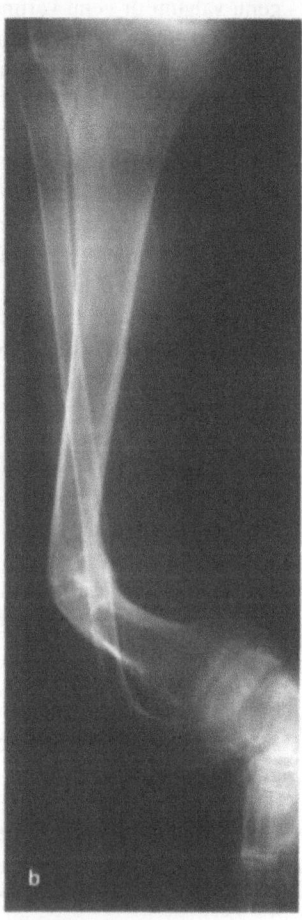

Pseudohypoparathyroidism

In pseudohypoparathyroidism, an X-linked dominant disorder, there is resistance to the action of PTH on the renal tubule. As a result plasma calcium is reduced causing tetany, and plasma phosphate is increased. Neither of the abnormalities is corrected by PTH administration. Additional features include a round face, short stature, cataract formation, mental retardation with calcification of the basal ganglion and short hands with short metacarpal bones, especially the fourth and fifth. Treatment is with the parent vitamin D, 50,000 to 200,000 units daily in order to increase calcium absorption or an appropriate dose of a shorter acting vitamin D preparation. Again, regular estimation of plasma calcium is necessary. The disease carries a good prognosis if treatment is started early to minimize the mental deterioration and cataract formation.

Cystinosis (Lignac–Fanconi Syndrome)

Cystinosis is a rare childhood disease transmitted as an autosomal recessive, in which there is deposition of cystine crystals throughout various tissues. The frequency is approximately one in 40,000 births. The exact mechanism appears to be an intracellular defect, possibly an enzyme deficiency, which allows the intracellular deposition of cystine crystals. The disease spectrum varies from severe extrarenal deposition and minor tubular defects, to severe tubular defects with minor extrarenal deposition. Unlike cystinuria, where there is a defect in tubular transport, the renal damage in cystinosis is non-specific. Microdissection studies have revealed a narrowing of the tubule adjacent to the glomerulus—the so-called 'swan neck deformity'. However, as this lesion is also found in other situations, e.g. congenital nephrotic syndrome, it may represent a secondary change. No gastrointestinal defects of amino acid transport have so far been described.

The disease presents in two ways. In the acute form the child presents with failure to thrive at around six months of age. He is lethargic and reluctant to feed, with polydipsia and polyuria. Generalized irritability and photophobia, due to cystine deposition in the eye, may occur. Urine testing reveals glycosuria, proteinuria and aminoaciduria. Death usually occurs from recurrent infections or severe metabolic derangements, e.g. acidosis or hypokalaemia.

The chronic form presents with vitamin D resistant rickets. Photophobia occurs and often hepatosplenomegaly secondary to cystine deposition. The characteristic urinary abnormalities are found and in the early stage renal function is well maintained. However, continuing cystine deposition in the renal interstitium and tubules leads to progressive interstitial fibrosis, and death from uraemia often occurs at 10 to 12 years of age.

The diagnosis is made by identifying cystine crystals in various tissues. Slit-lamp examination of the eye should be performed, and biopsy of either a lymph node or bone is helpful. Occasionally, crystals may be seen in peripheral white blood cells.

Both proximal and distal tubular functions are disordered. The majority of amino acids are excreted in the urine giving rise to an overall reduction in plasma amino acid levels. Renal glycosuria and phosphaturia occur. The distal tubular defects are an inability to concentrate the urine and an inability to acidify the urine, giving rise to systemic acidosis. Progressive interstitial fibrosis eventually decreases glomerular filtration and the features of uraemia appear.

Treatment is unsatisfactory and consists of treating complications, rather than the underlying abnormality. When rickets occurs it should be treated with large doses of vitamin D (or smaller doses of a more active compound) in a similar protocol to that used in vitamin D resistant rickets. If acidosis is severe, administration of sodium bicarbonate is necessary and potassium supplements should be given when there is hypokalaemia. When end stage renal failure occurs, renal transplantation may have good graft survival, but will not prevent the extrarenal features of the disease from progressing.

Galactosaemia

Galactosaemia is another rare disease presenting in childhood with the failure to thrive. Affected children have severe anorexia, cataracts, mental retardation and hepatomegaly. The disease is due to a deficiency of the enzyme galactose-1-phosphate uridyl transferase, leading to accumulation of a toxic compound, galactose-1-phosphate. This compound damages the renal tubule in a non-specific manner causing aminoaciduria, with characteristically low molecular weight amino acids such as serine, glycine and alanine being excreted. Galactosuria is also found due to the high plasma concentration of galactose but not renal glycosuria. Treatment consists of a galactose- and lactose-free diet, which produces a rapid clinical improvement.

Hepatolenticular Degeneration
(Wilson's Disease)

Wilson's disease is due to an error of copper metabolism and the patient is most likely to present with extrapyramidal signs. The defect is in the synthesis of caeruloplasmin allowing increased gastrointestinal copper absorption, and copper is deposited in brain, liver, eyes and kidney. Aminoaciduria occurs with threonine and cystine predominating, and occasionally glycosuria is found, but the other tubular defects are rare. The renal damage rarely causes major clinical abnormalities. Treatment consists of using the chelating agent D-penicillamine, which produces an improvement in the neurological and hepatic complications, but has little effect on the aminoaciduria.

Lowe's Syndrome
(Cerebro–Oculo–Renal Dystrophy)

Lowe's syndrome is an extremely rare inherited condition, usually present at birth, and consists of renal tubular defects, mental retardation and ocular defects, e.g. glaucoma and cataracts. In addition, there is failure to thrive and the development of renal rickets. The renal defect is a non-specific tubular damage similar to that of the Lignac–Fanconi syndrome. Treatment is directed at the complications rather than the underlying lesion, and is similar to that used in Lignac–Fanconi syndrome. However, the prognosis is extremely poor.

Acquired Adult Fanconi Syndrome

Adult Fanconi syndrome is a condition presenting with the symptoms and signs of osteomalacic bone disease, i.e. pain in the hips, shoulders and back, associated with muscular weakness and the classical 'waddling gait'. Typical radiographic changes of osteomalacia are usually found. There may be polyuria and occasionally muscular weakness due to hypokalaemia.

In addition to the generalized aminoaciduria, in which all amino acids are excreted but have normal or near normal plasma levels, there is renal glycosuria with a reduced Tmg. Plasma phosphate and uric acid are reduced due to increased renal clearance. There is also a defect in concentrating and acidifying ability. In some cases urinary potassium loss may be excessive.

The cause is unknown, but in 15 per cent of cases there is a family history, and it would appear to have an autosomal recessive inheritance pattern. Cystinosis does not occur in this lesion, unlike the Lignac–Fanconi syndrome. Treatment is again directed at the complications rather than the underlying disease. Osteomalacia is treated with vitamin D with good results and hypokalaemia with potassium supplements.

Other Causes

A number of drugs and heavy metal poisonings can cause renal tubular defects. The tubular defect is usually necrosis but isolated transport defects may occur. The most common of these, although rarely seen today, is the Fanconi syndrome which occurred with the use of outdated or degraded tetracycline. A similar syndrome may also occur with the use of parenteral neomycin. The antifungal agent amphotericin B often gives rise to renal tubular acidosis with severe hypokalaemia. Mercury ingestion also leads to tubular damage and Lysol and oxalic acid may also give rise to aminoaciduria and glycosuria.

Various isolated tubular defects have been reported in a number of other conditions. All the features of the Fanconi syndrome have occasionally been seen in patients with multiple myeloma, in which the damage is caused by reabsorption of Bence–Jones protein. Similarly, in patients with nephrotic syndrome, aminoaciduria and glycosuria will occasionally occur, possibly due to reabsorption of protein from the tubular lumen into the tubular cells. However, it may reflect tubular damage due to the original toxin causing the nephrotic syndrome. Aminoaciduria, renal tubular acidosis and polyuria have been reported in amyloidosis, and aminoaciduria may occur in patients with hyperglobulinaemia.

Idiopathic Hypercalciuria

A renal calcium leak has been found in some patients with idiopathic hypercalciuria (see Chapter 3).

Distal Tubular Disorders

Renal Tubular Acidosis

The kidney plays a major role in acid – base balance—to conserve bicarbonate and to excrete hydrogen ions. Approximately 85 per cent of bicarbonate is reabsorbed in the proximal tubule and the remainder in the distal tubule. The kinetics of bicarbonate reabsorption are similar to those of glucose and phosphate. Hydrogen ions are excreted, combined with ammonia to form ammonium (60 per cent) or as titratable acids (40 per cent). The ammonia is synthesized from glutamine in the tubular cells and phosphate forms the bulk of the titratable acid buffer substances. In acid urine there is increased excretion of ammonium and titratable acid, while the reverse occurs in an alkaline urine.

Hydrogen excretion occurs throughout the renal tubule, but the final process of urine acidification occurs in the distal tubule and collecting duct. Here, sodium is exchanged for hydrogen or potassium ions, the hydrogen being required to pass across an electro-chemical gradient. Normal subjects should be capable of acidifying urine to pH 5 or below. However, patients with renal tubular acidosis are unable to excrete urine with a pH less than 5.4 in the face of systemic acidosis. Patients with renal tubular acidosis may be divided into two groups: those with a proximal defect and those with a distal defect.

Proximal Renal Tubular Acidosis

Severe urinary bicarbonate loss occurs in a number of conditions in association with other proximal tubular defects. For example, patients with the Lignac–Fanconi syndrome, the adult Fanconi syndrome and more than 50 per cent of those with hyperglobulinaemia, due to either myeloma, cryoglobulinaemia or juvenile cirrhosis, have this form of renal tubular acidosis. The Tm for bicarbonate is reduced in this condition. Initially there is an alkaline urine, but as bicarbonate is persistently spilt and the patient becomes increasingly acidotic the distal tubule is able to reabsorb all the delivered bicarbonate. This occurs when the plasma bicarbonate is low, and the urine becomes acid again. Patients with proximal renal tubular acidosis usually have a greater degree of acidosis than those with the distal form.

Distal Renal Tubular Acidosis (Adult Form)

The adult form of distal tubular acidosis is the most common. It has a dominant inheritance with variable penetrance. The exact nature of the defect is unknown, but it results in an inability to establish a hydrogen ion gradient in the distal tubule with the retention of hydrogen ions. This gives rise to an alkaline urine and a systemic acidosis. In addition to the defect in hydrogen ion excretion, there is a slight bicarbonaturia and a reduction in ammonium excretion, the latter due to the relationship of ammonium excretion to urinary pH. Renal sodium and potassium loss also occur as a result of the acidification defect.

Other causes of distal renal tubular acidosis are nephrocalcinosis from hyperparathyroidism and hyperthyroidism, medullary sponge kidney, certain systemic disorders, e.g. Fabry's disease, Sjögren's disease, and amphotericin B therapy.

The disease usually presents in early adult life and is commoner in females than males, in a ratio of 2 : 1. There are four patterns of presentation:

1. Nephrocalcinosis. The patient may present with renal colic, and is subsequently found to have nephrocalcinosis. This is characteristically confined to the medulla but, when severe, will

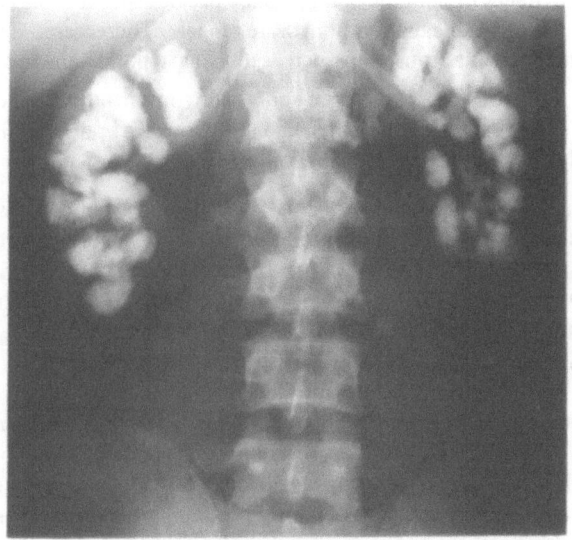

Figure 16. *Bilateral nephrocalcinosis in renal tubular acidosis.*

invade the whole kidney (Figure 16). Sometimes such calcification is found by coincidence during an investigation for unrelated symptoms. Nephrocalcinosis and renal calculus formation are due to an increased urinary calcium excretion and a decreased urinary citrate excretion in the presence of the acidosis; the latter favours the calcium phosphate precipitation. Calculi may lead to urinary tract obstruction, and secondary pyelonephritis occurs with recurrent urinary infection. There may be a reduction in GFR due to chronic pyelonephritis which makes the acidosis worse.

2. Bone pain, due to osteomalacia. Radiologically the lesions are identical to osteomalacia from other causes. The osteomalacia has been attributed to increased urinary calcium losses and to decreased plasma phosphate levels, the latter representing secondary hyperparathyroidism.

3. Attacks of periodic paralysis may occur, especially on waking or after a heavy carbohydrate meal. These are due to hypokalaemia, caused by increased urinary potassium loss.

4. Polyuria. This is due to an underlying concentrating defect and is exacerbated by the hypokalaemia. However, polyuria has an advantage in reducing the calculus formation.

The typical biochemical features are: serum sodium is usually normal; serum potassium is reduced and serum chloride increased (110 to 120 mmol/l); plasma bicarbonate is reduced (16 to 19 mmol/l); a random urine pH varies from 6 to 7 when the arterial pH varies from 7.3 to 7.35; and plasma calcium is usually normal or slightly reduced, as is plasma phosphate.

The diagnosis may be confirmed by an acidification test. It is not necessary to perform the three- or five-day test, but the short test of Wrong and Davies (1959) should be carried out. Ammonium chloride (0.1 g/kg of body weight in gelatine capsules) is given over 30 to 60 minutes at breakfast time and urine pH is measured hourly for the next five to six hours. A normal subject will acidify the urine to 5.3 or below, whereas a patient with renal tubular acidosis will not.

Treatment is to correct the acidosis with alkali and then the majority of the other complications and side effects will correct themselves. Usually sodium bicarbonate is given by itself or in combination with sodium citrate and potassium citrate. If sodium bicarbonate is given alone, plasma potassium levels must be monitored carefully and potassium supplements given as required. Vitamin D should not be administered for two reasons: first, the osteomalacia will improve and heal with correction of the acidosis, and second, vitamin D will increase urinary calcium excretion, making the nephrocalcinosis worse.

Distal Renal Tubular Acidosis in Infants

The infantile form of renal tubular acidosis is rarely seen today. Unlike its adult counterpart, which is a chronic disease requiring long-term therapy, the infantile form presents as an acute illness, and with appropriate treatment the renal tubular defect is reversible. The disease, which is commoner in males, is not inherited and the cause is unknown.

The condition usually appears between the ages of 12 and 18 months and presents as failure to thrive, with constipation, apathy, hypotonicity and marked dehydration. The biochemical findings are similar to those in the adult except that plasma potassium and phosphate are usually normal, and in approximately 50 per cent of the children the blood urea is raised due to dehydration. Nephrocalcinosis is present in some children but rickets does not usually occur.

Treatment consists of correcting the sodium deficiency and acidosis with intravenous infusions of alkali such as sodium lactate. When the child has improved and will take oral therapy, sodium citrate or sodium bicarbonate solution is given for up to 12 months. Treatment is then reduced slowly with careful biochemical monitoring to ensure that the acidosis does not recur.

Nephrogenic Diabetes Insipidus

Nephrogenic diabetes insipidus is a rare hereditary condition in which there is an abnormal insensitivity of the distal tubular cells to the action of vasopressin (antidiuretic hormone, ADH). The posterior pituitary gland is anatomically and hormonally intact and ADH is found in the blood and urine of affected individuals.

The condition presents with polyuria, leading to episodes of acute volume depletion which may be exacerbated by other fluid losses, e.g. vomiting and diarrhoea. Mental and physical retardation has been reported in some children but this may be due to repeated episodes of severe dehydration. Bilateral hydronephrosis is also found as a result of the large urine volumes. The diagnosis is confirmed by a standard eight-hour dehydration test which results in weight loss and no increase in urine osmolality. Urine osmolality does not improve with the administration of vasopressin.

When there is acute dehydration, intravenous fluids are required to restore the extracellular fluid volume. Long-term therapy consists of a chlorothiazide diuretic and a reduced salt intake. This produces a mild degree of volume contraction with increased sodium and water reabsorption in the proximal tubule, and decreased fluid delivery to the distal tubule producing a reduction in urine volume.

Acquired Lesions

A defect in the concentrating mechanism leading to polyuria is common in a number of metabolic states. In hypercalcaemia there is an inability to achieve an increased medullary osmolality, possibly due to a defect in sodium transport in the loop of Henle. Similarly, in hypokalaemia the medullary osmolality is reduced, possibly because of impaired sodium transport in the loop of Henle or impaired water reabsorption in the collecting duct. Lithium intoxication is also associated with nephrogenic diabetes insipidus.

Miscellaneous Conditions

There are three disorders of sodium metabolism whose aetiology is not fully established. However, as a possible transport defect in the renal tubule is postulated, they merit consideration.

Bartter's Syndrome

Bartter's syndrome is characterized by hypokalaemia with normal or low blood pressure and raised plasma renin and aldosterone levels. On renal biopsy patients have hypertrophy of the juxta-glomerular apparatus. It is postulated that there is a decrease in sodium reabsorption by the proximal tubule which gives rise to volume contraction. This causes a compensatory rise in plasma renin and aldosterone in order to increase sodium reabsorption from the distal tubule and consequently increased potassium loss occurs from the distal tubule. Treatment is potassium replacement.

Gordon's Syndrome

Gordon's syndrome is characterized by hypertension and hyperkalaemia. Plasma renin and aldosterone levels are low. The hypertension is due to the increase in extracellular fluid volume induced by an increase in proximal tubular sodium reabsorption. The increased extracellular fluid volume decreases plasma renin and plasma aldosterone, which in turn reduces potassium secretion in the distal tubule. Treatment consists of diuretics and a low salt intake.

Liddle's Syndrome

Liddle's syndrome is characterized by hypertension, hypo-kalaemia and reduced aldosterone levels. It is postulated that the underlying mechanism is an increase in distal tubular sodium reabsorption, giving rise to an increase in extracellular fluid volume leading to hypertension and low aldosterone levels. The low potassium level is regarded as a secondary effect of the increased sodium reabsorption. Treatment is a low sodium diet and the diuretic triamterene, which blocks sodium reabsorption in the distal tubule.

References

Chapter 2

Boulton-Jones, M., *Acute and Chronic Renal Failure* (Topic Pack Series), Update Books, London, 1980.

Hodson, C. J., Maling, T. M. J., McManamon, P. J. and Lewis, M. G., The pathogenesis of reflux nephropathy, *Br. J. Radiol.*, 1975, suppl. 13.

Chapter 4

Wrong, O. and Davies, G. E. F., The excretion of acid in renal disease, *Quart. J. Med. N.S.*, 1959, **28**, 259.

Further Reading

Chapter 1

Asscher, A. W., Urinary tract infection in women, in *Recent Advances in Nephrology*, N. F. Jones (Ed.), Churchill Livingstone, Edinburgh and London, 1975.

Asscher, A. W. and Brumfitt, W. (Eds), Symposium on urinary tract infection, *Kidney Internat.*, 1975, suppl. 4.

Bailey, R. R., The relationship of vesicoureteric reflux to urinary tract infection and chronic pyelonephritis—reflux nephropathy, *Clin. Nephrol.*, 1973, **1**, 132.

Bailey, R. R., Roberts, A. P., Gower, P. E. and De Wardner, H. E., Prevention of urinary tract infection with low dose nitrofurantoin, *Lancet*, 1971, **i**, 1112.

Freeman, R. B. et al., Long-term therapy for chronic bacteriuria in men, *Ann. Int. Med.*, 1975, **83**, 133.

Winterborn, M. H., The management of urinary infection in children, *Br. J. Hosp. Med.*, 1977, **17**, 453.

Zinner, S. H. and Kass, E. H., Long-term follow up of bacteriuria of pregnancy, *New Engl. J. Med.*, 1971, **285**, 820.

Chapter 2

Cove-Smith, J. R. and Knapp, M. S., Analgesic nephropathy: an important cause of chronic renal failure, *Quart. J. Med. N.S.*, 1978, **47**, 49.

Gower, P. E., A prospective study of patients with radiological pyelonephritis, papillary necrosis and obstructive atrophy, *Quart. J. Med. N.S.*, 1976, **45**, 315.

Heptinstall, R. H., The enigma of chronic pyelonephritis, *J. Infect. Dis.*, 1969, **120**, 104.

Heptinstall, R. H., Pyelonephritis: pathologic features, in *Pathology of the Kidney*, Little, Brown and Co., Boston, 1974.

Hollander, W. and Blythe, W. B., Nephropathy of potassium depletion in *Diseases of the Kidney*, M. B. Strauss and L. G. Welt (Eds), Little, Brown and Co., Boston, 1971.

Chapter 3

Coe, F. L. and Kavalich, A. G., Hypercalciuria and hyperuricosuria in patients with calcium nephrolithiasis, *New. Engl. J. Med.*, 1974, **291**, 1344.

Crawhall, J. and Watts, R. W. E., Cystinuria, *Am. J. Med.*, 1968, **45**, 736.

Guttman, A. B., Uric acid lithiasis, *Am. J. Med.*, 1968, **45**, 756.

Pak, C. Y., Urolithiasis, *Kidney Internat.*, 1978, **13**, 5.

Pak, C. Y., Ohata, M., Lawrence, E. C. and Snyder, W., The hypercalciurias: causes, parathyroid functions and diagnostic criteria, *J. Clin. Invest.*, 1974, **54**, 387.

Chapter 4

Dent, C. E. and Stamp, T. C. B., Hypophosphataemia osteomalacia presenting in adults, *Quart. J. Med. N.S.*, 1971, **40**, 303.

Lee, D. N. M., Drinkard, J. P., Rosen, V. J. and Gonick, H. C., The adult Fanconi syndrome, *Medicine (Baltimore)*, 1972, **51**, 107.

Morris, R. C., Sebastian, A. and McSherry, E., Renal acidosis, *Kidney Internat.*, 1972, **1**, 322.

Seegmiller, J. E., Friedman, T., Harrison, H. E., Wong, V. and Schneider, J. A., Cystinsosis, *Ann. Int. Med.*, 1968, **68**, 883.

Index